SLIM BY SUGGESTION™

ABOUT THE AUTHORS

Roz Collier, co-founder of the Slim by Suggestion programme, is an experienced lecturer and trainer. She is also a qualified teacher, clinical hypnotherapist and stress management counsellor.

Georgia Foster is a highly experienced therapist, having trained in the UK, USA and Australia. Co-founder of the Slim by Suggestion programme, she is a lecturer, personal development trainer and clinical hypnotherapist.

slim by
Suggestion™

10 EASY STEPS TO WEIGHT LOSS WITHOUT WILLPOWER!

Roz Collier & Georgia Foster

Thorsons

Thorsons
An Imprint of HarperCollins*Publishers*
77–85 Fulham Palace Road
Hammersmith, London W6 8JB

The Thorsons website is www.thorsons.com

and *Thorsons*

are trademarks of
HarperCollins*Publishers* Limited

Published by Thorsons 2001

10 9 8 7 6 5 4 3 2 1

Slim by Suggestion™ is a trademark
of Roz Collier and Georgia Foster

A catalogue record for this book
is available from the British Library

ISBN 0–00–712666–2

Printed and bound in Great Britain by
Martins The Printers Limited, Berwick upon Tweed

Contents

ACKNOWLEDGEMENTS

Our thanks to all participants on the Slim by Suggestion workshops for their warmth and feedback, and especially for proving to us, through their successes, that the mind tools from the workshops really, really work.

We would particularly like to thank Helen Craven of The Craven Clinic, Hammersmith, London, and Amanda Seyderhelm, of ReadytoWrite.com, our very own literary agent.

Roz

I would like to thank Jim and Gill Davies, my wonderful parents, Lee, friend and best therapist, my sister Carol, Andrew and many friends for their unwavering support and their faith in Slim By Suggestion, and to Georgia, good friend well met.

Georgia

I would like to thank my Nana, Georgina Foster, for being British, which enabled me to study and work legally in the UK. I would also like to thank Aldeburgh, Suffolk, for the precious time we had developing and writing this book away from the hustle and bustle of London life.

My mum, Bev, dad, Richard, and sister, Virginia – I can't thank you enough for your long-distance support and belief in me.

Roz, my business partner and motivator – thank you for all your personal and professional support, especially your wonderful editing ability.

Thanks to Joy, the Pownell family and the Clark family for providing me with a roof over my head, which gave me the stability to continue to build my business.

Thanks to Oan, Sal, Sue, Fiona, Janet, Helen, Fi Fi Lamour, Hazel, Louise, Kirsty and Kath for keeping me up when I had too many things to do. Thanks to all my friends in Melbourne and London who have been with me through literally thick and thin.

1
Setting the Scene

Here is an extract from Sarah's diary:

Friday: I'm really excited. I've just bought this *Slim by Suggestion* book. I've heard it's a really good book to help me lose weight. I'm not sure how it works but a colleague has lost loads of weight and said I should just start reading it, as it will all unfold. Sounds great. Let's see how I go. I'll make Monday the day to start. I suppose I could start reading the book now, although maybe I will make this my last weekend before I knuckle down to being healthy. This time I just know it will work. If she can do it, so can I.

Saturday: Writing this in bed as I went to a party this evening. Guess what? It was a total disaster as I ate all the tuna dip. It wasn't until this really attractive guy called John (who I really like) made the comment, 'Would you like some hummus for main course now?' that I realized. I went *so* red. Then I went to the bathroom and tried to make myself sick. He will never like me because I'm just a fat frump. I felt so awful that I left, saying I had a headache. My friend Sandra, who's pencil thin, says I always seem to have a headache when we go out these days. The truth is that I can't stand being around slim people. Everybody is slim except me. I can't wait for Monday when I'll be able to start the Slim by Suggestion programme and get slim once and for all.

Why isn't there a miracle drug I can take to make the fat just melt away? I feel so depressed and unattractive. Now I'm exhausted with it all. I'm lying in bed writing this damn sad diary, lonely and fat. I can't believe I ate all that bloody tuna dip. I can feel it adding to my hips and my legs. My stomach feels like a beach ball.

Sunday morning: I woke up and instantly remembered what John said to me last night. He'll never like me. I've completely ruined it now. In fact, no one is ever going to like me. What's the point of being slim? I'll be just as lonely as I am now. What an idiot I am. If people really knew my thoughts they would think I was mad anyway, and I probably wouldn't have any friends either.

I'm dreading the family lunch today. Grandma is coming and I know what's going to happen. First thing she'll do is remind me that the reason I don't have a boyfriend is because I'm a 'career girl'. I must say, I'm starting to agree with her. Maybe I should be more like my friend Mary, who's a housewife. She's got all the time in the world to work out. If I was a housewife, I'd have no excuse but to be slim. Yes, life would be so much easier.

Sunday evening: I was right. Everybody in my family was looking at my body and how much weight I've put on. I feel like my head is splitting with all these thoughts running around. What's wrong with me? I've eaten everything in sight, drunk too much wine and now I'm in my lovely flat and I feel like getting totally out of it with food and wine. I'm dreading tomorrow at work. I'm not even sure I'll be able to fit into my clothes after my horrendous binge weekend.

Anyway, be positive! Tomorrow is a new day and I'm looking forward to reading the book that will change my life.

Monday: I left the book at home! I'm so hopeless and stupid. How am I ever going to lose weight? I feel grumpy and angry with myself. This morning I was standing in a really full train and all I could do was look at the other passengers to see who was thinner than me. There was one girl in a beautiful suit, very slim, but it's OK – she was ugly. A woman asked me if I wanted a seat. Oh my god, she actually thought I was pregnant! I felt so awful I just wanted to cry except I had to get off at the next stop. Now that has to be a sign – I am seriously fat. I wished I could just go home and sleep through this nightmare and never ever see anybody again.

When I finally arrived at work, Mum called to say she is worried about me. She thinks I'm over-aggressive and that I seem angry all the time. I felt like saying to her, if you had a body like mine, wouldn't you be? I can't talk to her about my weight because I know what she'll say – just eat a little less and exercise a bit more darling, it works for me. Maybe the book is just another con, just another depressing diet.

Tuesday: I had a very busy day today, and as I had a bit of a hangover this morning, I had to have some good stodge for breakfast to get over it. I can feel the rolls of fat under my bra. I feel so uncomfortable. How can I ever possibly lose weight? It's just too hard.

And to cap it all, my boss pulled me into the office. I just knew something was wrong. He said there had been a complaint made about me. I was surprised at the time, although after the phone call with my mother, perhaps everything is getting to me. Perhaps I'm just an aggressive, negative person anyway. He said he supported me but felt there was some cause for concern. When he asked me if everything was all right, personally, I just broke down and cried. And, of course, once I start crying I can't stop, and I couldn't even speak a language that was intelligible. So they sent me home.

I feel awful, totally undignified and just a hopeless mess. I think I need a holiday. Yeah, right, get out in your bikini, Sarah, and see how good you feel! I can't possibly take a holiday until I lose weight because it'll be a waste of time and money. And I've just bought a book and haven't even bothered to open it. I bet it's like all the others, just some impossible diet. I don't know why I bother. Even thinking about dieting has made me want to go into the fridge, and you know what, I might as well. I haven't eaten anything for ages and nothing's going to work.

Wednesday: I've just got home. Work was OK, but now I'm having an anxiety attack because my ex from two years ago has phoned to say he's in town for the weekend and can we catch up. I'm beside myself. The last time he saw me I was at least $1\frac{1}{2}$ stone lighter. He will just think I've turned into a complete mess. He has a new girlfriend who's a model! I can't possibly see him.

I can't believe I'm saying this. I'm 35 years of age, OK job, OK home, OK friends. I should have got over this weight business by now. I'll just have a snack to keep me going and I'll settle down to start that book...

Sarah is just one of the millions of people who talk to themselves. You can understand from her diary how talking to herself in this way makes her feel as if she is going crazy. She is obsessed with losing weight and focuses on it all the time. Her thoughts are accompanied by her constant internal chatter, which keeps up a running commentary on what she is, but mostly isn't, doing.

People with weight issues think about their physical weight constantly.

It's not at all uncommon to wake up in the morning and immediately start to think about what you will be able to eat. Everything can revolve around how you will be able to deal with the day, what you will be able to eat and what everyone else will think of you.

Why We Are Writing This Book

This book is written for anybody who has problems around food, who talks to themselves about food, and for anybody who feels their eating is out of control just some of the time or all of the time. If you eat when you are not hungry, you are feeding yourself for other reasons, and this book will provide you with the insights you need in order to change, forever, your relationship with food.

The book is based on the successful eight-week programme (and weekend workshops) called Slim by Suggestion™. Participants attend an evening session once a week for the eight-week period. Each session deals with a particular topic, and in between sessions they will listen to a CD track, keep a food diary and an emotional journal. It is due to the fantastic feedback and encouragement from the participants that this book has been written. Case studies which accompany each chapter represent real people with real problems, although names and details are changed, and are included in order that you, the reader, can understand that many, many people share the emotional turmoil of being overweight and/or out of control with their eating. One of the course participants made this statement at the end of the programme: 'Slim by Suggestion is the emotionally intelligent way to become slim and stay slim.' Another said, 'The biggest influence on my eating habits since my mother!' Our aim is to bring the programme to you in your own home.

How to Use This Book

The Slim by Suggestion programme consists of 10 easy steps. These are described in detail in Chapter 7. Before you begin the 10-step programme, however, you must read Chapters 1 to 6 and, as soon as possible, listen to Track 1 on the accompanying CD. Do this once or twice daily until you start the programme at Chapter 7, when you will move on to Track 2. You will be asked to listen to that track once or twice a day for six to seven days. Then you will move on to Chapter 8, where there are further instructions.

The CD contains all the instructions you will need and is an important part of the progress you will make. It may sound ridiculous that listening to a CD for 20 minutes twice daily will change your behaviour around food, but it does. The CD is about releasing old negative thought processes that you have created and stored in your unconscious mind. We explain more about this in Chapter 5.

Most people who try dieting do so by using their willpower (their conscious mind). They tell themselves that if they could only stick to the diet, exercise more and be strong, they would lose weight. Willpower dieters will recognize the internal conflict that going on a diet provokes, and those unhealthy and unsupportive inner voices which literally feed that emotional conflict: 'I don't know why I'm even buying another diet book. Look what happened the last time – I put on even more weight. I'm such a failure at everything. Dieting's not going to work ...' This is why all diets fail. They ignore the fact that food is a symptom, not a cause.

Slim by Suggestion takes a new approach to becoming slim and staying slim.

It helps you to understand issues of emotional conflict, so that you can re-programme the unconscious part of your mind and change your inner dialogue to provide supportive messages. The result is that you gain control over eating behaviour and consequently lose the emotional and physical weight you have been carrying around.

The Authors' Personal Experiences

We thought it might be helpful for us to share with you our own personal experiences with weight.

GEORGIA FOSTER

I was brought up the traditional Australian way – home in the suburbs, pool in the back garden, summer holidays at the beach. I can't remember why I started to gain weight consciously at around 12 years of age. I was a shy child but generally happy-go-lucky, with two loving parents who worked hard at keeping home a warm and safe place to be. My sister and I had everything a child could really want.

When I hit puberty, I started to gain weight. I also began to notice that what you looked like mattered in order to fit into a group. This was the early 1970s when people were becoming body conscious and magazines started to feature 'dieting' regularly. None of my friends had a weight issue and I felt very isolated and alone. The way to deal with this was to overeat, to secretly eat, and eat so much that I would feel sick. Then I could not sleep at night due to the guilt about what I had done to myself. I am not sure whether it was obvious to many people but I know that it was a concern to my parents, who felt that the more they focused on it the more I would eat. They were right there.

I remember once listening to a family member suggest that it was just puppy fat and that I would get over it. I was mortified that people were talking about me and scared that they appeared so concerned. So I ate more.

I had one friend in whom I secretly confided. She was bulimic. I could never have stuck my fingers down my throat but she could, and we often overate together with absolute glee. I also had friends who overate and seemed never to put on weight.

I had a crush on one of my sister's boyfriend's friends when I was 14. I was, as usual, plump and unhappy with my body. I have always been motivated to achieve many things (except to manage my weight) so I worked part-time from 14 so I that I would be independent. I suspect the busier I was, the less time I had to think about me, really. I worked in a 24-hour supermarket and really enjoyed it. I felt very adult. It was also the place where I used to eat everything in sight (paid for, of course). The man I had a crush on used to pick me up and take me home, where everybody would be sitting around watching the late night movie. He once said to me as I was reaching for my hundredth piece of chocolate, 'Georgia, can you afford to eat that?' I looked very dumbly at him but, knowing exactly what he meant, I answered, 'Of course I can. I earned it, I paid for it.' He said, 'Georgia, you know what I'm saying. Can you really afford to eat that chocolate?' I was so embarrassed as this personal comment was in front of my parents, my sister, her boyfriend and some other people. I was so humiliated, I just wanted to cry. He then went on to explain to me that if I lost weight I would be kind of attractive!

That comment has stayed with me forever. Comments like that were really hurtful, and the only way I could deal with them was to overeat. Some people would have gone the other way and chosen not to eat, but I was a feisty girl who, when told to do white, would do black. So I just got fatter, fatter and fatter.

I regularly went on diets that worked for a week and then put the weight back on along with a few additional pounds. Over the years, with more and more examples of failure to my credit, my self-esteem dwindled. This was not apparent on the outside, as I was very good at hiding it. We all have examples of when people have wounded us. I have included them here not to suggest that I live in the past but to demonstrate by examples in the book that being wounded is real and truly hurtful. The examples are to illustrate the power of words and how they, for no particular reason, burrow right into our mind.

It took me many years, from my late 20s into my 30s, to finally deal with my weight. The principle that food is the symptom not the cause is very true. What I didn't realize was that my low self-esteem stopped me from ever really using my full potential. I lived in a shell of anger, frustration and fat! I loathed myself and truly believed I was not worthy to be happy and, especially, to be slim. It took many years of bad relationships, binge eating and crazy dieting to finally understand that there is a way through and out of the situation.

I truly want you to understand that I have been there, and I never want to go back. In fact, with the skills honed via lecturing for Slim by Suggestion, I don't have the ability to go back. It took me 30-odd years to find the right answer for me. I hope that by reading this book and listening to the CD I can save you 30 years!

ROZ COLLIER

I was always the sporty type and was very fit and lean until my mid-20s, when things went pear-shaped, literally. The beginning of my own rocky road was when I left home and flat-shared. Looking back, I had no idea about what to eat or portion size. My eating became very haphazard. Half the time I couldn't be bothered, and the other half of the time I was eating too much. I didn't make a commitment to a regular eating routine, but as I was swimming regularly, attending aerobics classes and rushing about, there was no effect at that time on my size.

As my career developed, I found I was lunching a lot and drinking a lot. Pressure of work and moving to London meant that the exercise got left behind. I didn't really have the time, with all the long working hours, the socializing and pubbing. I was a 'ladette', keeping up with the boys pint for pint, eating man-size meals and generally acting like a glutton.

So at around the age of 23, I decided to take up an aerobics class as I was getting unfit, short of breath and fatter. This was to be a defining moment in my life as I joined a class and immediately sustained a sports injury. That was me ... all or nothing ... had to be competitive ... had to work harder ... jump higher, and of course, I went at the exercises in the class as if I was still fit and didn't listen to my body telling me I was pushing it too far, too fast. So I struggled on, being propped up by an osteopath for more than 10 years, just to keep me going so that I could still work and do well in my career.

The type of injury I had caused pain in my back, thighs and shins. And it doesn't go away. To deal with it you can either fill yourself with painkillers or take time off to rest and heal. NO WAY! A perfectionist can't take time off from their career. They are as dependent on their professional life as the person with low self-esteem who covers it up by defining themselves by their job role, by being valuable at their workplace. So I struggled on. Instead of pills I discovered that lager seemed to help the pain go away and food in general seemed very good at helping me deal with the stress I was creating for myself. I was at an all-time low by 30. Bloated-looking, two sizes bigger than my natural body size, binge-eating, binge-drinking, incapable of relaxing or being calm, miserable in my marriage and totally stressed out at work. I may have appeared confident to other people but my confidence was just about non-existent.

So I got a divorce and I was so truly miserable that I dropped the two dress sizes by the misery diet. Not to be recommended. It just shows how little I was taking care of myself physically and emotionally, and I just lost interest in food. Once I was living on my own, however, I began to establish a routine of eating little portions of healthy food. I didn't feel as though I was on a diet, more like my body was self-regulating down to my natural weight.

So I was happier with my body and my confidence began to rise. It was then, however, that I realized the underlying difficulties were still there. As I got happier, I began to go back to my old binges. It was through training in stress management and clinical hypnotherapy that I understood how I was using food and drink to suppress my stress. I was lucky that I was motivated to undertake training as it opened the door for me to gain control over my thinking and therefore my eating and drinking. It's a great pleasure to be able to pass on those skills and experience on the Slim by Suggestion programme and to know that there really is a way to be normal around food.

Setting the Scene

2

Inner Dialogue

Millions of us talk to ourselves, and millions of us talk to ourselves like Sarah does in her diary (*see Chapter 1*). In fact, most of us say things internally that we would never, ever, verbalize to another person, or even dream of saying to our worst enemy. At Slim by Suggestion, we call these internal conversations Inner Dialogue. When a person wants to make a change, such as eating healthily in order to get in shape, this will trigger an even more intense bout of self-talk. When you talk to yourself, do you use any of the following statements, or something similar?

- 'You'll never keep the weight off anyway.'
- 'Since when have you been successful at losing weight? You're just a failure.'
- 'Why bother!'
- 'Who do you think you are, thinking you deserve to like your own body?'
- 'People will just say, there you go again, on another diet. I wonder how long this one will last.'

- 'Some chance! You're getting a bit over-confident, even thinking the programme is going to work. You know what you're like!'
- 'You think you can trick yourself using a CD to program the unconscious mind. Well *you* can't. I know everything about you. I know how you think and feel, and I don't believe anything is going to work for *you*.'
- 'How can it possibly work when you're so pathetic and out of control?'
- 'You can't even get started. That's how useless you are.'
- 'Go on – one more can't possibly make you any fatter.'
- 'It's never going to work for you, so you might as well put it off till tomorrow.'

We call this particular voice The Inner Critic. It is strong, strident and opinionated. There's a test at the end of this chapter (*see page 23*) for you to rate the strength of your Inner Critic. Sarah, our diarist, joined the evening programme and discovered the extent to which her strong Inner Critic was ruling her life. The voice was real and so strong that, like many people, she was in fear of its negative comments and really believed its opinions were true. Every time she wanted to do something, her Inner Critic would voice its opinion and she would instantly believe that she didn't have it in her to succeed in whatever she wanted to achieve.

The Inner Dialogue Theory

We are born with a unique personality and a mind that is set up to protect the personality and physical body in whichever way it can. In order to be emotionally and physically protected, a child will develop defensive armour, which will protect them from being vulnerable. As we are developing, for instance, we discover that our parents like certain aspects of us more than others. They like and reward the smiling child, the fun child, the child that is nice and quiet and so on. And so we develop 'parts' to our personality. We can deliberately bring out the 'part' of ourselves that parents and/or other people like best, and the parts that get us love, like the comic part, the acting part, the sporty part of ourselves. So what naturally happens is that certain parts which may not be acceptable to others, such as the creative part, the demanding part or the inquisitive part, may well become suppressed – hidden away. Those parts of ourselves that do not get positive feedback and reward are therefore held in check so we don't show or experience our original and whole personality. These parts 'cannot' be revealed, as they will make you feel vulnerable and unacceptable, like when you were a child, so they lie dormant as far as possible. The challenge we all face, however, is the fact that all parts want to have equal expression.

For instance, if your parents wanted you to be a lawyer and your great dream was to be a fashion designer, in most people the creative 'fashion designer' part will be suppressed. Years later, sitting in your legal practice, you will know and feel that it's just not right and something is missing. We often forget all about the original creative part as it is so suppressed; however, it will always be seeking an outlet – you may find yourself doodling pictures and designs. The Inner Critic will leap on this activity: 'What are you doing? That doodling is a real waste of time. What would people think if they could see you now?' Then you feel miserable and guilty, and you don't even know why, but you do know from experience that you can feel better if you eat something, usually a lot of something, or have a good session on the booze.

There are many voices to your internal dialogue. We will concentrate on The Inner Critic, The Perfectionist and The Pleaser, which are like the border patrol or the cops patrolling between the 'good' and acceptable parts and those 'bad' parts that have been suppressed. Their job is to stop you expressing those parts that will make you feel vulnerable, even though the vulnerability only applied when you were a developing personality and just an innocent and immature child.

This type of statement is one we have heard many times: 'When I feel like bingeing it's as though a part of me just wants to eat everything in sight. It's like a self-destructive inner demon that simply takes over my whole personality, and the more I try to avoid this demon the stronger it becomes. Afterwards, when I've eaten everything in sight, I feel so depressed, so out of control and guilty. If people knew what I'm like, I'm sure they would think there was something seriously wrong with me. It's as though I have a split personality. Every other area of my life is in control except this urge.'

This is a typical scenario for a person with a strong Inner Critic. The emotion of vulnerability or fear of abandonment will trigger a bingeing session. Then after the fridge is completely raided, The Inner Critic steps in to tell you once more how hopeless and disgusting you are. Your Inner Critic has now got another example, unconsciously, of when and how you have failed.

Anybody who has had a bingeing experience can recognize that while they are in the bingeing state they feel as if they are not in control; the bingeing part is in total control. The Inner Critic will then remind you about this behaviour, again and again, which will lower your self-esteem (even more) and can lead to bouts of depression.

> This Inner Critic's voice can be so strong that we sometimes think we are going mad.

In Sarah's case, she began to differentiate between her own voice and the voice of her Inner Critic. She started to hear just how hard on herself and almost cruel this voice had become. When you listen to The Inner Critic for a long time, it is understandable that you think it is your own voice, your own personality, and it is not. It's just the voice of your Inner Critic, one part of you, not all of you. By thinking through the information about this voice and listening to her CD (Track 1), Sarah quickly realized that by acknowledging it she could begin to recognize the difference between it and her real voice; she also began to recognize the different tones of voice of her other (defensive) parts.

Often The Inner Critic is the most vocal of the inner voices, especially when we would like to make a change or move forward. If an attempt at change has been unsuccessful in the past, it will provide you with every example of your past failures; and if there isn't an example, it will make up a scenario of future worry or a hypothetical failure example anyway. The Inner Critic was created by your mind to help protect you from vulnerability; however, it has become too good at its job and has taken over. The Inner Critic can't let you succeed because it will be made redundant! That is its fear. Now you can reassure your Inner Critic that it is a valuable part of your Inner Dialogue because it has a role to protect you and to allow you to consider what is right and wrong for you. You can begin to observe and negotiate with your Inner Critic, acknowledge its voice and its concerns. The recommendation is that you don't suppress this inner voice but start a dialogue with it.

RULES OF AN INNER CRITIC

1. It knows everything about you so it can always remind you of all the times you have lied, cheated, contemplated awful actions and thought terrible things! It knows when you have strange sexual thoughts, when you have wanted to be vicious to someone, when you did something shameful.

2. It always lets you know when you have failed.
3. It supports anybody who criticizes you by saying 'I told you so'.
4. Its voice is always there when you want to make a change.
5. The Inner Critic tells you that you are not as good as someone else; it loves to compare and contrast.
6. The Inner Critic makes sure that you won't lose weight because you have already failed before. The Inner Critic has already decided that you won't be able to cope with failure. It can't allow you to experience failure as it is too painful.
7. The Inner Critic loves to use props to support its case against you. Have you got a talking mirror? Get up tomorrow morning and look in the mirror – it starts to talk to you: 'You look so crap, I don't know why you bothered to get up'; 'Good grief, it's going to take hours to put your face on'; 'Well, it's obvious you overate yesterday, there's pounds more on your cheeks'. And there are talking scales: 'You could break these scales, you've put on pounds'; 'I don't know why you're looking at the scales, you already know you're hopelessly overweight'; 'So you thought you'd lost some weight. Fat chance!'; 'It looks like you've lost a couple of pounds ... you've just worn the scales out and it's reading a wrong measure'.
8. THE ROLE OF THE INNER CRITIC IS TO CRITICIZE AND NOTHING ELSE.

TEST YOUR INNER CRITIC!

Write down your answers to the following questions:

1. What aspirations did you have as a child to be special, different to everybody else?
2. In which areas do you remember being perceived as ordinary?
3. What does the critic like to criticize about your body?
4. Do you have talking scales? What do they say to you?
5. Do you have talking mirrors? What do they say?
6. What do you think you are good at?
7. What does your Inner Critic say to you when you decide to lose weight?

At this stage your Inner Critic will be going into overdrive. This is very beneficial as you will hear it in its true colours. It will be feeling totally threatened by what you have read, as the backbone of The Inner Critic is fear. It is based on fear. It is also worried about what other people will think of you. That is why, on the Slim by Suggestion programme, we recommend that you don't tell anyone about the fact that you are reading a book and listening to a CD to help you deal with weight issues. (Tell everyone when you are successful and no sooner!) This is due to the fact that your Inner Critic loves to compare and contrast you with other people – and there may well be people around you who do not want you to succeed as it will make them feel vulnerable! So they will try to sabotage you, offer you food, manipulate you into an eating occasion you don't want, take you out drinking (lots of lovely calories) and generally be secretly unsupportive.

Look out for the saboteurs around you.

The Inner Critic is a voice based on habit. If you have been on 'diets' before, you will need to manoeuvre around the Critic, so this time you are on a 'healthy eating programme', as it is not the same as a (punitive) diet. We recommend that all your self-talk discusses healthy living, such as healthy eating and exercise, and avoids old words like 'diet' and 'weight problems/issues'. Breaking the pattern of your internal dialogue begins the process of successful change. After all, that is what you want to achieve – the normality of eating healthily so that you can become your natural body shape, and exercising regularly so you are toned and invigorated.

The wonderful thing about the Inner Dialogue theory is that you will come to discover another voice within. At the moment it is too shy or too suppressed to come forward. That part is the slim part, the part that likes to be slim and the part that knows you have the ability to be slim. The slim part is there, and we can know this by one simple fact: you would not have bothered to go and buy this book if that slim part were not within you. Even in the past, when you may have tried hundreds of diets, you would not have bothered to attempt to get slimmer if you didn't have that slim part within.

> This book is all about how to introduce the slim part into your daily life, and how to bring its support and positive intent and helpful dialogue to the forefront of your mind.

However strong and strident your Inner Critic is, remember that it is frightened and fearful now, and finding out its fears is a great start to your new negotiation with this voice. You need to be able to have a dialogue with it so that you can do and be what you want. Writing down any Inner Critic self-statements is a good start. Laughing at what it is saying is also good; observe and listen to it. You don't have to be it; you can begin to be yourself.

The Inner Critic says: How can listening to a CD and reading a book allow you to lose weight?

You: What are you frightened of?

The Inner Critic: I am frightened you will fail and about what people will think.

You: Well, I thank you for your concerns and I am sure you have a good reason for this feeling from past experience. However, I am going to try the book out. I'm going to try it for a few days and see how I go. We can keep on talking like this from now on.

The Inner Critic: Let's see how long you last. I'll give you less than a week. I'm really worried that other people will be saying: 'There you go again, another faddy diet thing, and it won't make any difference.'

You: Yes, you're right, people may be thinking that, but no one will know I am on this programme, only you and I do. So unless someone is a mind-reader, how will they know? Whenever I'm in public, I will eat healthily. No one needs to know. In fact, it is no one else's business. Thanks for your concern but I am going to succeed on this programme with the help of my slim part, which is only supportive.

Remember, never agree with your Inner Critic when you have a dialogue. Put an alternative, any alternative, into the conversation, even if you don't believe it at first. If you agree with The Inner Critic, you have taken on the Critic role and it only knows how to criticize. Now, just ask yourself this question: what is your favourite part of your body? Now are you saying that The Inner Critic does not exist?

Claire's Story

Claire, 38, has been married for 12 years and has two children. Claire has been a yo-yo dieter for as long as she can remember. When she dieted for her wedding and reached her target weight successfully in record time, she had a definite goal and it was worth it (she starved herself on a very low-calorie diet which made her feel totally deprived). Claire recalled how much she felt in control and confident, sexy and alive.

After the wedding she went back to work for a number of years. She gained weight, lost it, gained it, lost it. It was a general pattern. Her Inner Critic always reminded her that being slim would not last and that she would be on this yo-yo dieting track for the rest of her life. The Inner Critic also told her that her husband had promised to love her for better or worse, so let's see what worse 'really is'. Claire listened to The Inner Critic, and once she had children, the weight piled on. Her self-esteem started to get very low and her marriage began to fall apart. In these situations, we can only report one side of the story and Claire's was quite sad. She had married someone who was not a great communicator. He provided for the family and worked hard and never really commented on her weight, but her Inner Critic did it for her. 'He really thinks you're hopeless, that you can't succeed at anything. He finds you sexually unattractive. He only comes home to you now for the children.'

When Claire recognized that this was the voice of her Inner Critic, not her husband (no one can read someone else's mind accurately), she started to see that what she was doing around food created that self-fulfilling prophecy. She believed The Inner Critic, and while she was in thrall to her Inner Critic, she could not have high self-esteem. Building her self-esteem through the CD helped her to see that being more confident meant she was better company. She recognized that she didn't need to be so miserable all the time. Her husband commented on how bright she was. This had a domino effect on her relationship with her children as well.

Self-worth is the most wonderful gift you can give yourself, and by challenging The Inner Critic you can have high self-worth and self-esteem. Claire started to notice that she didn't need to eat that second piece of cheese and that, instead of avoiding spending time with her husband by hiding and snacking in the kitchen, she began to enjoy his company, and that food didn't have the same impact because it only fed The Inner Critic. Her Inner Critic, as she now knows, was stopping her from having high self-esteem and from feeling that she deserved to be happy. The nicest statement came from her husband. He said 'I thought I had lost her for life, but she is back again. I didn't realize she had gone until she came back.'

Remember, you will not stop The Inner Critic from talking but you can talk with it and negotiate with it to disempower it. It is just one part, one voice, not all of you.

RATING YOUR INNER CRITIC

Look at the following statements and see how they apply to you. If your answer is 'rarely', score (1); for 'sometimes', score (3); and for 'frequently', score (5). Add up your scores at the end and consult the key below for your personal Inner Critic score.

Questions	1/3/5
1. I wake up at night worried about yesterday.	1
2. I replay conversations after I've had them to see what I've done wrong.	1
3. I don't like the way my clothes look on me.	5
4. When I'm with other people, I wonder if they're critical of me.	3
5. I'm cautious about trying anything new because I'm afraid of looking stupid.	1
6. I'm afraid people will laugh at me and I'll be humiliated.	1
7. I worry about what other people think.	3
8. I feel inferior to other people.	3
9. I wish I had more self-control around food.	5
10. When I look in the mirror, I check to see what's wrong with me.	1
11. When I read over something I've just written, I'm not satisfied with it.	1
12. I'm afraid there's something fundamentally wrong with me.	1
13. I worry about what people would think of me if they really knew what I was like underneath.	1
14. I compare myself with other people.	1
15. I seem to attract negative people.	3
16. I question my decisions after I have made them and think that I might have done better.	3
17. When I say 'No' I feel guilty.	5
18. When I fill in a questionnaire like this, I'm sure that I won't do as well as everyone else.	1
19. I avoid taking risks if I can help it.	3
20. When I think about self-improvement, I feel that it is a lost cause.	3

Inner Dialogue

Key

If you scored 20–44, your Inner Critic is weak.

If you scored 45–74, your Inner Critic is medium.

If you scored 75 or above, your Inner Critic is strong.

SOME THINGS TO TRY

- Get to know the difference between your voice and the voice of your Inner Critic. Acknowledge The Inner Critic – start a dialogue with it rather than attempting to suppress it. 'Thanks for your comments, and for bringing your concerns to my attention. I will consider what you have said before I take action.' Laughing at what it says, and writing down any Inner Critic statements, are also good ways to differentiate between you and your inner voices.
- You need not tackle The Inner Critic head on. Just changing your self-talk to 'healthy-eating programme', 'healthy living', 'reducing excess body fat' will begin to break old patterns.
- Always put an alternative to your Inner Critic. Don't fall into its trap and agree with what it says!
- Recognizing that your voice and the voice of The Inner Critic are different allows you to start to hear the 'slim part', and other supportive parts of your personality. You don't need constant negative commentary, so discover your real voice using all the techniques in this chapter.

Slim by Suggestion

3
The Perfectionist

The Perfectionist is a very powerful inner voice. It is a controlling, restricting, vocal part of you, which you can experience as a strong energy. Working in tandem with The Inner Critic, it has to do a 'perfect' job in preventing you from being vulnerable.

At this very moment, you may be saying to yourself some or all of the following: 'Why are we going to talk about a part that is a perfectionist? What does it have to do with me?'

- 'I can't be a perfectionist as I am overweight, I struggle with my weight and I am either on a diet or constantly thinking about it.'
- 'If I was a perfectionist, I would be able to manage my eating and drinking, I'd be at an exercise class every week and I would always be able to fit into my clothes.'
- 'There is no way I am a perfectionist. I'd be in control of my life and my eating if I was.'
- 'People who know me would laugh if I said I was a perfectionist.'

The Perfectionist's voice directs you to behaviour and actions which will be viewed by you and everybody else as 'perfect'. Or you won't attempt them.

Your Perfectionist will only allow you to try things it knows you will do 100-per-cent right – in your daily life, your work, your home life and in your behaviour and relationships.

On the plus side, your Perfectionist will have got you to where you are today. If there are things you are proud of, you can be sure that your Perfectionist allowed you to attempt them and provided a lot of drive and energy for you to achieve and succeed. However, a Perfectionist part cannot possibly allow you to start something that may cause you to stumble or fall flat on your face. That would make you just too vulnerable.

If one of your suppressed parts from childhood is a desire and ability to be really good with languages, then your Perfectionist will attempt to keep that part suppressed so you won't be vulnerable. As an adult, when you think about attending an evening class in Spanish, your Inner Critic and Perfectionist will conspire to stop you going.

- 'No one in your family has ever been any good with languages,' says The Inner Critic.
- 'The amount of time and effort you will have to put in to learning to speak Spanish will only distract you from the really important things, like your job ... who else leaves the office before 6pm?' says The Perfectionist.
- 'It's not as if you know you have any language talent. Anyway, if you want to learn something, why don't you do a course that would be useful in your career, like another qualification in XXXXXXXXX?'

- 'You must be a bit crazy to want to learn Spanish. Who will look after your children as well as you can? If you go to the class, then your mother, husband or babysitter will be responsible for them – is it really worth the effort?'

This is typical of the type of dialogue from The Perfectionist – it sounds reasonable, logical and often has a quiet, powerful, authoritarian tone of voice. So our pertinent question is, 'When was the last time you lost weight and kept it off successfully?' We don't recommend that you ponder over the answer too much as your Inner Critic is probably saying something rude or obnoxious to you! Tell your Inner Critic that even if the answer is 'never' at the moment, you have a new strategy, thank you!

Your Perfectionist has to succeed, and if it does not have a successful example of losing weight and maintaining that body size and image, it will not allow you to even attempt a 'diet' programme. Its ultimate purpose is for you to give 100 per cent and to achieve 100-per-cent success in anything you do. So it will say, 'You can't show me any proof that you can lose weight, so let's not go there!' And that is why people who struggle with their weight find it so hard to even get started on a weight-loss programme – you will have to wait for conditions to be 100-per-cent 'right' before you can start; it will have to be the 'perfect' type of diet regime, the best one you can find which fits in with your lifestyle, and so on. And so the start date gets put back, your Inner Critic beats you up and you are so miserable that you eat the fridge.

You can make a start, and it begins with new dialogue and negotiation with your Perfectionist – right now! Just like the new conversations with your Inner Critic in Chapter 2, start to consider what that Perfectionist part is saying. You can also start by saying, 'OK, this is not a new "diet". I have decided from now to reduce my excess body fat, so all I am going to do is eat healthily and exercise a bit more – and I intend to do that to the best of my (our!) ability.' There is a lot of support for you on the CD, particularly Track 1 at this stage.

The Perfectionist part can be very strong yet beneficial in other areas of your life. For example, if you have struggled with your weight you, in all probability, excel in other areas of your life. Good at making friends? Successful in your job? Perhaps you have a very successful hobby or you are a great host. The Inner Critic and Perfectionist will support these activities because they know you are successful and talented in these areas. They support the parts that are 'good' and acceptable.

Understanding and negotiating with The Inner Critic and The Perfectionist will mean that you can start to recognize that they are just voices, not your personality, and that they have been holding you back from having good self-esteem and preventing your Slim part from having a voice and an influence.

Through listening to Track 1 on the CD, The Perfectionist will start to understand that you have examples of success and so it will feel safe for you to achieve your slim you. With the examples of slim success you are creating in your mind, The Perfectionist will know how to support you in getting there and how it feels to be a success at eating healthily and losing excess body fat.

CAN YOU RECOGNIZE THE PERFECTIONIST IN YOURSELF?

- Do you try and do everything yourself – as no one will be able to do the job as well as you?
- Can you recognize that you never start things you feel you may not be able to complete or achieve? Do you prevaricate?
- Do you criticize people who leave things half-finished?

- Are you judgmental about other people when they are scruffy or sloppy, tatty or tarty? 'If only he/she paid more attention to detail'; 'They would look good if only they had clean nails, shoes, better haircut etc.'; 'She's really letting herself down – she's being so loud everyone's looking'.
- Do you get embarrassed for other people?
- Do you have (strange) rules/rituals – everything in one kitchen drawer being just so? Or certain procedures that you have to do in a certain order when you are involved in a task?
- Do you make lists or pride yourself on your orderliness?
- Do you have judgemental internal conversations? 'They can't possibly get that done, doing it that way'; 'Be interesting to see how they manage that – they haven't got the right people in to do the job for a start'.
- Are you tempted to interfere with other people's activities? Would you take a paintbrush off someone so you can do it 'properly'?
- Do you feel frustrated when you watch someone performing a task? Could you do it better/faster/neater/more cleverly?

Sometimes, without knowing it, we choose something that we aren't good at to make us socially acceptable. How many of us have looked at a successful businessman, happily married, clever, handsome, and thought, there's got to be something wrong with him? How can X or Y be so 'perfect'? There is something in our society and upbringing, and supported by our Inner dialogue, which gives us the notion that we can't be perfect or too successful. The Perfectionist won't let you start something unless you can succeed and your Inner Critic says you can't be good at everything.

So the compromise, even if you are not aware of it consciously, is that if you want to be successful, that's fine, but something has got to make you human. So there is always the weight business. How many people do you know who yo-yo diet, can't keep to one suit or dress size, who binge eat and/or drink and yet who appear very organized and successful?

How many times have we judged or criticized someone who 'has everything'? Society makes us judgemental. 'There must be something wrong with her. Maybe she had a bad childhood, or maybe she's secretly unhappy'; 'I bet he's not well-endowed' ... there is no need to go on with these less than lovely judgements!

If you are too good, says The Inner Critic, then be really good at not losing weight; be perfect at not losing weight; that way you get to be a normal human. Meanwhile your Perfectionist won't even let you start.

Rebecca's Story

Rebecca had acknowledged that her Inner Critic and Perfectionist were very vocal. When it was explained to the group how vicious and ruthless The Inner Critic could be, she looked completely terrified and extremely uncomfortable. She also recognized how very manipulative The Perfectionist can be.

Rebecca's reaction is typical. For many people who have a particularly strong Inner Critic and Perfectionist, it can be too scary to contemplate life without these inner voices and the emotional security blanket they provide. Rebecca told me later that the scariest thing about acknowledging The Perfectionist was that now she would have to lose weight! She felt that, finally, she had found a tool that showed her a way through her negative self-doubt and prevarication about losing weight.

This frightened her as there was a contradiction – the thought of not being able to succeed at losing weight was actually a place, which on some level allowed her to feel safe. Rebecca had some real fear feelings and her own dialogue was something like, 'Oh s***! I've been found out. I've allowed The Perfectionist to keep me overweight – but do I really want (the challenge) to be slim?'

She spent some time, using her emotional journal (see Chapter 7), thinking about that challenge, and on reflection she recognized that The Perfectionist was actually being supportive as she didn't have a successful example of being slim. So she did not know how to get there. And as we know, The Perfectionist will not allow you to do anything unless it has a successful example to work with.

By listening to Track 1 on the CD, Rebecca installed successful outcomes of being slim in her mind so that her Perfectionist could understand that it was safe to be slim. Rebecca noticed that as she negotiated with and recognized her Perfectionist behaviours, she became much more 'light-hearted' and less stressed out. She loved the concept of being excellent at things, rather than perfect. She said that trying to be really good or excellent was actually achievable, and in fact the state of 'perfection' could only last a nanosecond before something would change. The group loved it!

Helena's Story

Helena was a classic Perfectionist. She had a high-powered job, a totally organized life and was in complete charge of her financial and emotional affairs. She had a happy relationship and yet was, and had been, consistently two stone overweight. Helena was a very intelligent woman who was good at balancing everything except her weight.

Over the course of The Perfectionist evening session and during the following week, Helena discovered that her Perfectionist part was controlling her life. This meant that she could never relax and allow things to go wrong. She realized that she was very intolerant of people who were unable to 'deliver 'on time. Helena was able to acknowledge that whatever people 'delivered' to her never seemed good enough, and even if it was their best effort, she would always find fault. This led Helena to experience total frustration. She would be stressed and impatient, and then she would push down these feelings by overeating.

Helena started to recognize that not everybody saw the scenario the same way as she did. Or should we say that when she acknowledged her Perfectionist was totally scared of failure, she knew why it was impossible for her to delegate. She also began to understand a huge intolerance she had towards people who were 'feeble and pathetic'. She could now see that she was totally unable to deal with people who were 'sick', and especially 'off sick' from work. Her Perfectionist had never allowed her to take time off from work, even when she had needed a rest to recover. Perfectionists can't be ill as it is not physically perfect. Helena was typical in this respect as people who have a high Perfectionist have a tendency to neglect themselves physically.

In the same way, she understood she could not lose weight because her Perfectionist was too fearful of failure. She began to see that her Perfectionist needed to recognize that not everything can go her way, and that worrying about how it 'should have been' was keeping her very highly stressed. Helena began to negotiate with The Perfectionist and to make changes. She was and is much happier and more easy-going. She says herself that she is never going to be a laid-back person, but that is OK, as she has now and will continue to have success with her weight both physically and emotionally.

Julie's Story

Julie was working part-time and had a couple of children at home. After The Perfectionist section of the programme, she announced to the group that there was no way she could be a Perfectionist or have a Perfectionist part. She just couldn't agree that it related to her in any way.

In group debate the following week, the discussion focused on feeding children. Julie mentioned that she would only feed her children fresh food and that she would never provide microwave or frozen meals; meals had to be fresh. The group's view was that there were times when convenience foods were necessary. Julie became rather agitated about this 'cutting corners' and the group began to laugh. Julie saw the funny side as the group said 'I'm not a Perfectionist then!' Several other examples came up over the next couple of weeks and Julie was finally able to recognize and challenge her Perfectionist.

She spent time thinking about her behaviour and found that this part existed and had a huge influence on her. Its voice was so strong that she realized it was the reason she described herself as having been a 'terrible prevaricator'. It also explained why she never ventured into a long-term healthy-eating programme to lose weight because her Inner Dialogue would not let her fail in anything. Julie really enjoyed the course and felt that it had helped her life in so many ways, not least of which she was really proud when she lost her first stone of excess body fat.

What Happens to Anorexics?

Some of you may know someone who is an anorexic, or you may even be one yourself. A full-blown anorexic is a total perfectionist in the eating part of their life – they can starve themselves perfectly. Their Inner Dialogue is mainly with their very strong Perfectionist, and they will not, or are unable to, negotiate with it. Their Perfectionist has always been demonstrably 100-per-cent right and effective. This is how an anorexic and their Perfectionist part can ensure the other aspects of their life seem less vulnerable and disappointing – one area is totally perfect.

An anorexic's Perfectionist can specialize in not eating, and as a result the anorexic has the support and considerable energy of their Perfectionist part. For those of you who are not anorexic but have periods when you have that tendency, it will be when aspects of your life are not going the way your Perfectionist wants. As a result, it will need to assert control in some way to make you feel in control of something, and not totally vulnerable. If this applies to you, using negotiation and Track 1 on the CD will be beneficial.

The Perfectionist's Confusion

The behaviour of an anorexic clearly demonstrates that they have very few, if any, parts of their life that they feel they have control over; yet they are potentially extremely high achievers. It is the same for most of us, but to a much lesser degree. When many people start Slim by Suggestion, they will say, 'I was really good last week – I hardy ate anything'. This is the voice of The Perfectionist (who is naturally attempting to achieve the aims of the programme, i.e. lose excess body fat, in a couple of days). And there will be a tendency for high Perfectionists with strong Inner Critics to initially fluctuate between not eating at all and binge eating. This shows clearly how there is a conflict between parts. The Inner Critic observes The Perfectionist and the confusion of behaviours and says, 'What can you do properly?'

Learning to Love Your Perfectionist

All the Inner Dialogue parts have responsibilities and voices. You can parent all of them and negotiate with them. You can metaphorically embrace them by understanding that each holds valid opinions and by having a supportive but firm Inner Dialogue with them. Once you communicate with the different voices, you can get some balance in your life. Start to listen to what is really going on, and listen to Track 1 on the CD.

SOME THINGS TO TRY

Sometimes we need to challenge our Perfectionist and differentiate between it and The Inner Critic. A good way to start is to make a list of the things you are not particularly good at, such as sport, cards, writing letters, cooking, public speaking, meeting people, having and expressing an opinion. Try to write down at least 15 things that you are not particularly good at; listen to what your dialogue is saying! When you have compiled your list, ask yourself, have I actually ever tried any of the things on my list? How do I know I'm not good at them?

If your Perfectionist hasn't let you try something before, you will need to counter its dialogue and your behaviour, so try to do something new that you haven't done or attempted before. For instance, read a short book on a subject you know little about, but interests you. Take the time to watch something obscure on television or investigate that hobby. Do something for you that is not work-related or for other people. Chapter 4 has more on the topic of other people.

Positively, and under your direction, your Perfectionist can be a great and supportive part, enabling you to achieve so much and to enjoy your leisure time. This is another characteristic of The Perfectionist – if you are a career person or raising children, you will find it difficult to even think about LEISURE! (The perfect picnic, the perfect house, the perfect golf swing, the perfect holiday. Need we go on...) There are potentially so many parts that were suppressed as a child, and to have the opportunity to expand these into your life is something achievable. That includes reducing excess body fat and finding an interest in some form of physical exercise.

4
The Pleaser

The Pleaser is the third part of the triumvirate that creates the protective border patrol between the acceptable parts of you and those parts that you suppressed as a child.

> The Pleaser can be a forceful voice with manipulative power. It represents the part of your personality that makes sure everybody else is all right.

It has to make sure that everybody else comes first. One could think that this is a traditional part for women but it can be equally strong in men.

Has someone ever invited you to dinner, or to a social event, and you really don't want to go, but before you can gather your thoughts to refuse the offer politely, you hear this little voice saying 'Yes'. I can't believe I said that! That is your Pleaser talking for you.

People who have a strong Pleaser will never be able to get their needs met. If you get what you want, that means you are being too selfish. The Pleaser part is constantly worrying about what other people think of you.

It is very scared of you not being liked and so a Pleaser will go 100-per-cent out of their way to make someone feel comfortable, to the detriment of their own time and comfort. There is naturally a strong connection between The Pleaser and The Perfectionist, supported by your Inner Critic.

A Pleaser will have lots of friends and will be likable and lovable. It is often the case that The Pleaser is so busy feeding everybody else, physically and emotionally, that they have little time for themselves, if any. Spending time with you means less time with others. One of our concerns about maintaining a strong Pleaser is that while your needs are not being met, the only safe way to achieve some sort of personal satisfaction is through food. Somehow this seems to be an acceptable trade-off because your belief is that YOU have to make sure everybody is being fed somehow, whether physically or emotionally.

The Pleaser will usually be a very good cook, have wonderful dinner parties, put on an over-the-top buffet, cook the best breakfast, as all these are ways you can 'feed' everybody else. By being sociable, playing counsellor or confidante to others, you and your Pleaser can be feeding them; and as you go out of your way to please others, you will be feeding your own needs too.

After the guests have left, however, or while you are doing the dishes, the leftovers go straight into your mouth. Why? Because you have not allowed any time for yourself as you were pleasing and nurturing others yet again. The internal conflict will start – 'Did anybody ask me how I was?' The Pleaser can and will answer that for you: 'You can't put your needs first. People will think you are selfish and unfeeling. Remember, if you don't focus on them, they may find out that you are so incredibly self-centred. You'll lose all your friends!'

The inevitable reaction to a strong Pleaser dialogue like this is to push the fear away and keep the vulnerability hidden – some people can literally 'clothe' themselves in a protective barrier of excess body fat. This is at the extreme end of the spectrum, but one of the things that does keep The Pleaser quiet is to feed it. That and going along with what it says, like 'Yes' when you mean 'No', and, of course, continuing to look after everybody else's needs ahead of your own.

Be careful, because The Inner Critic will probably pop in here now if it hasn't already to remind you how much time you are spending with yourself reading this book – and to The Pleaser that means you are letting someone else down. The Inner Critic will be supportive because The Pleaser is characteristically so worried about everything that it gives an ongoing stream of dialogue that the Inner Critic can totally agree with – keeping you from moving forward. It thinks it is keeping you safe.

After hosting a dinner party, for example, The Inner Critic will run a dialogue around in your head such as this one: 'What did I say?'; 'Did I offend someone last night?'; 'I drank too much, I'm sure I offended someone'; 'So and so didn't look too happy when they left'; 'I'm sure it was a mistake to put X and Y near each other, I really thought they would get on'.

You may churn over and over different things you could have done or said, thinking how much more you could have done to please everyone. The Pleaser part within goes completely crazy, rewinding and fast-forwarding like a video trying to find some incident where you could have been more nurturing or more understanding. Ideally, you should have tried to solve everyone's total emotional problems. Then, when someone who came to the party phones to thank you, instantly you feel they are going to criticize you, either for your chocolate mousse, your other party guests or basically how crap you are as a host or hostess.

The Pleaser

Characteristics of The Pleaser

If you have the inability to say the word 'no', then you have a very strong Pleaser.

People who cannot say 'no' are just too concerned that they will hurt someone, and as a result that person won't love them anymore. One of The Pleaser's biggest personality traits is fear of rejection. So begin to ask yourself questions like, why is it so important for this person to like me? Does it really matter? What would happen if I did say 'no'? Would they still be a friend?

It can also be a wonderful attribute to be a Pleaser. People love Pleaser-type people because they always know that there is someone there to listen to them. They always know that there is someone who will give them unconditional love and attention. However, The Pleaser will demonstrate exhaustion in sighing, sleeping a lot to avoid dealing with people, and retreat into illness as an opt-out to dealing with other people. The Pleaser will generally have the trait of being a hypochondriac – being sick or ill is the only way they can get some sort of 'authorized' attention. The unheard Inner Dialogue will be 'Hello, I'm here. Look after me like I've been looking after you. Now it is my turn.'

One of the ways in which you can find out whether you have a Pleaser-type personality is to keep an Emotional Journal (*see Chapter 7*) and include how often you are sick and whether your illness is one that allows you to have more attention than your Pleaser would normally allow. Because The Pleaser is exhausted and needs to rest, illness becomes the only safe option. Nothing else is as effective as an illness. 'That will really make them think. What would they do without me?'

The Pleaser may seem weak in nature, but be assured that a Pleaser part can be so strong that an individual may go a whole lifetime and never really know what they want and who they really are.

The Pleaser character may well drink too much, as well as eat too much. They feel that they have to be sociable because saying 'no' to a social event is rejecting someone. A Pleaser will have a very busy social life and a lot of friends (whether they are genuine is another thing). Playing the saint can be very rewarding but it becomes tiring, boring and incredibly frustrating to know that all you are doing is looking after everybody else.

The Pleaser is well known for being sexually active. How can one possibly say 'no' to sex?

We are not suggesting this means being sexually open to all, but an underlying thought is 'If I don't say "yes" they may go and have an affair'; 'They may reject me'; 'They will think I don't love them'.

What about asking for what you want sexually? Do you often sacrifice your own sexual needs to please your partner? Does spending time having your needs met sexually make you feel incredibly uncomfortable because you are taking up too much time? Meanwhile, your Inner Critic is saying horrifying things about your thighs, penis size, big breasts, crap technique, cellulite etc. The Pleaser's response to this is to do everything to keep your partner happy, and so what if you don't get any pleasure or satisfaction.

The Pleaser will always be apologizing for everything. 'I'm really sorry about the size of my bum or beer belly'; 'I'm really sorry that the meal wasn't perfect'; 'I bet you've had better boiled rice than this'. Some of this is to create an opportunity for you to receive some attention or compliments so that you are given feedback and praise. You have to remember that The Perfectionist is aligned to this and will support these inner conversations along with The Inner Critic: 'You are just not good enough'. No wonder a big Pleaser part goes hand-in-hand with low self-esteem.

THE PROBLEMATIC PLEASER PART

The problem with having a strong Pleaser is that there is a constant Inner Dialogue going on, such as, 'Why am I doing this? Don't they realize I need to be heard? I'm tired of this game'. A Pleaser-type personality will assume that other people can read their mind. They can get into a habit of overeating and getting very angry and depressed that nobody loves them for themselves. If this goes on too long, The Pleaser can cause a complete breakdown. If this happens, you will cry, feel incredibly helpless and useless, and eat everything in sight, not for an hour or a day, but for weeks.

An exhausted person, through an overactive Pleaser supported by The Perfectionist and The Inner Critic, will want to hide from the world and be a hermit. If they can't hide away, they may as well just overeat. Then the excess body fat will protect them and prevent them from interacting with the world. Ultimately, The Inner Critic is the strongest voice, and it will not let you go out because you are such a mess. A Pleaser character will find it difficult, if not impossible, to take responsibility for themselves because they are too busy pleasing.

The person with a strong Pleaser will have low self-esteem because they do not spend any time on themselves. Often, people reflect back to us that they don't actually know who they are and are frightened of who is really inside. 'If they knew how apathetic I was, they wouldn't like me'; 'I wouldn't have any friends because I'm so weak'. In fact, this is The Inner Critic speaking. It likes to keep you in a fear state and it loves supporting The Pleaser because it makes you feel totally useless, boring and uneventful. You need other people's lives to make your life interesting, don't you?

The Pleaser also has some great attributes. Having a Pleaser as a friend is wonderful, but any healthy relationship needs healthy dialogue and a Pleaser can rarely express what they want. By listening to Track 1 on the CD you will start to be more assertive and proactive about what you want.

Slim by Suggestion

PLEASER HEALTH WARNING

We must warn you though: some people may not like it when you become more like yourself and less like a Pleaser. Your best friend, your partner, your work colleague may be sabotaging you and manipulating you for their own gain and to have their needs met. Pleasers have a lot of hangers-on, so be prepared for some backlash. Friends, if they are true, will accept the changes you need to make and will continue to make. The ones that don't ... well, you will begin to see them in their true colours.

BULIMICS AND THE PLEASER

Those of you who are bulimic will have a very strong Pleaser. A common reaction to its strength and control is to severely overeat. If you are always pleasing other people, there is a high chance that you will regularly stuff yourself with food. Pleasers look upon their bingeing with disgust. They usually feel totally revolted and embarrassed that they have this habit of overeating. It is an 'out of control' energy by which The Pleaser demonstrates its power and strength. Please recognize that it is just a part, and on some level it is protecting you and helping you to deal with life. The Pleaser's Inner Dialogue can often make you panic and cause you to be chronically over-anxious; then the overeating helps you fill the inadequacies that your Inner Critic thinks you have. Overeating is not a sin; it is simply the way The Pleaser operates in order to get its needs met.

Do You Recognize The Pleaser?

- Do you feel the need to make sure everybody likes you?
- Do you feel uncomfortable if you put yourself first?
- How do you feel when people don't acknowledge what you have done for them? How do you feel when others don't say 'thank you' when you have invested a lot of personal and emotional effort?
- When you wake in the mornings, do you feel a sense of disappointment that you haven't baked that cake for Granny, even though Granny doesn't even know you were thinking about baking that cake?
- Do you feel guilty if you don't say 'yes' to everything that is asked of you?
- Do you wake up in the mornings feeling guilty about what you said last night, and that they might not talk to you ever again?
- Do you panic thinking you didn't say enough or do enough for someone? If you had done something more for that person, why did they not love you more?
- Do you feel the need to regularly satisfy your partner sexually, even though your own sexual needs are not often met?

Judith's Story

Judith had quite a chuckle to herself when we discussed The Pleaser. She resonated with The Pleaser completely and was extremely vocal during this part of the programme.

She was in a traditional family role and did all the domestic chores for her husband and two adult sons. She was about four stone overweight. She discussed the fact that she cooked big meals because she had three men to look after, so she ate what they ate.

All meal times were carefully planned to make sure they had all the right healthy foods. Her sons, one 18 and the other 24, were still living at home, and Judith did everything for them. It is possible to think that perhaps they were lazy and unhelpful, but when you have a Pleaser the size of Judith's, then even if they had offered or begun to help, her Pleaser would instantly tell her that she was not doing enough for them.

Judith had created a definite no-win situation for the family dynamics. I suggested to her that perhaps she could practise being more assertive with herself in one part of her life that didn't involve her family. She couldn't find an area in which she believed it would be possible! So we did a bit of brainstorming in the group, and with a lot of laughs, we discovered that she could be more assertive while shopping. Judith said she couldn't even return something that was mouldy to a shop in case she offended the assistant. So she agreed that she would be more assertive and less pleasing when she was on her own. She felt that practising with strangers was easier for her than with her family.

She used Track 1 on the CD twice a day and reported back to the group the next week that 'it works!' We were all delighted at her results. She explained that, amazingly, the perfect opportunity arose the next day. She went to her local supermarket where the cashier short-changed her. She knew it as she walked away, and questioned whether or not to say something. She took her chance to make a difference and turned around to explain to the cashier that he had short-changed her. He looked at her and then the receipt and apologized. She said her face was flushed and her heart was pounding, and she was concerned that he would make a mockery of her. When she left she felt alive and in control.

Some of you may think this was trivial, but if you have a strong Pleaser part then it can be a milestone. Once you start to take baby steps towards being assertive, and by listening to Track 1 on the CD, it will start to become a habit to say 'no' when you truly want to. It just takes practice. The mind will soon learn that this is how you now think and respond to situations.

Jackie's Story

Jackie had the strongest Pleaser we had met. She was totally at everybody's beck and call. She stayed late in the office to do other people's work, and felt she needed to keep her mobile phone on – even during our sessions and at the weekends – just in case someone needed her. She worked for a very demanding boss and it was assumed that she would clear up any messes made by others. Jackie was tired all of the time and, once home, would eat whatever was in the fridge till she was completely stuffed. She was miserable.

Jackie also looked after her elderly mother. When I asked her when was the last time she had a holiday, she scanned her mind and said when she was a teenager. She is now 40! She is a classic case of 'If I stop and think about what my needs are, people will think I'm selfish. If I ask myself what my needs are, they might be too frightening. So I have to avoid myself and keep looking after everybody else.'

The thought of being able to say 'no' was really terrifying to her and, unfortunately, she must have felt that it was all too much to deal with. We never saw her again.

The Pleaser Theory

The Inner Dialogue theory is a powerful one, and the dialogue and behaviour of these parts can be powerful too. The Pleaser is probably the most self-destructive of these parts because the underlying factor will be anger. If you have a strong Pleaser and you do not get your needs met, you will have to resort to anger to interrupt your experiences. This means stuffing your face, and probably blaming everybody else for making you suffer.

Once you are in control of your Pleaser, however, you will be able to acknowledge it as a quality and not a hindrance. You will also have to acknowledge that it is a case of 'once a Pleaser, always a Pleaser', but the secret is that it doesn't control your life and it doesn't have the power over you to make you devote yourself to other people. It is very beneficial to recognize that it is OK to please people but not at the expense of your own time, your own happiness and your wellbeing.

A Pleaser does have some wonderful attributes. What would a mother be without unconditional love? What would a friend be without dropping everything when it really matters? A healthy Pleaser is fine, as long as it doesn't lower your self-worth and self-esteem and then lead to overeating, self-abuse and ANGER! Nobody deserves to be angry; it leads to unhappiness, depression and, ultimately, disease. We discuss anger in Chapter 11.

By getting in touch with your Pleaser, you will start to become able to say the word 'no'. We know it is difficult; please trust us, we have been there. By listening to Track 1 on the CD, you will start to learn that you have the ability to break the pattern. A Pleaser will always have a lovely pleasing part, but the more you are assertive, the better your life will be.

SOME THINGS TO TRY

- Each week, think of one aspect of your life in which you want to become more confident. Plan it in advance; make sure you write it down somewhere as well.
- Think about a situation in which someone is controlling your space, where you are allowing this person to control you. Think about situations where you feel you are being taken for granted.
- Be aware that if you have a strong Pleaser, saying 'no' will be a bit of a shock both for you and the recipient, but there are ways of doing this. Constructing a dialogue in your mind and practising saying what you want is a really valuable tool. No one said it would be comfortable; what change is comfortable? Go with it because once you say 'no' you will feel a bit guilty, a bit odd and definitely vulnerable. Think about it. Do you feel guilty and angry when you say 'yes' anyway?
- Practise saying what you want to say, out loud or in your mind. Whether it is to the woman at the make-up counter who insists you try a perfume you know is already giving you a headache, or to Aunt Mary when she offers you another slice of cake. Aunt Mary may not like it, but would you have liked yourself if you had eaten the cake?
- Try and make a habit of doing one thing to 'please yourself' every day. Spend that 15 minutes reading a magazine or a book. Listen to something you want to on CD or radio. Wake up in the morning and say 'What can my Pleaser part do to please me today?'

5
About Your Brain

Now that you have been listening to the different voices of your Inner Dialogue and negotiating with them, you will be allowing positive and motivating dialogue to be heard and receiving support from your 'slim' part. You will have been listening to Track 1 on the CD and letting those 20 minutes, once or ideally twice a day, give you relaxation and the benefits gained from the release of any build-up of stress chemicals. You will have experienced what can be called self-hypnosis, or self-induced relaxation, just by listening. At the beginning of the book, we said that the CD is an important part of the progress you will make on the Slim by Suggestion programme; this chapter will explain why and also the reasons why it is so important to get in control of your thinking and your Inner Dialogue.

There are two sides to the brain: the right brain – the unconscious mind – and the left brain – the conscious mind. They perform different functions and have different attributes.

The messages contained on the CD are specifically designed to work on the unconscious mind, where all the old unwanted habits, beliefs and behavioural triggers are stored.

On the CD the language, the tone of voice and the repetition of the messages are to facilitate communication with the unconscious, which is why the voices sound different to the way we speak when we communicate consciously.

The Conscious Mind

Described as the left brain, the functioning of your conscious mind is exactly that – you are aware of its activities consciously. It is logical in its thinking; it works in a way that is sequential and step by step. It uses words and is where your Inner Dialogue is created. The conscious mind is aware of past, present and future and is concerned with time. It is under the control of the unconscious mind, in that the defences of the unconscious, for instance the activities of The Inner Critic, Perfectionist and Pleaser, will manifest themselves into conscious activity. That activity may take the form of inner voices or a conscious stream of thoughts and dialogue that will prevent you from moving forward and being vulnerable. We will look at the patterns of thought that are 'excuses' later in the chapter – they are a prevalent type of conscious thinking activity that can be lumped under the heading of protective or negative thinking. Equally, the conscious mind can provide positive thinking and activity; it doesn't matter to the conscious mind what your thinking and Inner Dialogue is as long as it protects you from experiencing vulnerability.

We are not aware of many aspects of ourselves until we consider them consciously. If I ask you to think about your elbow, or your big toe, you will immediately focus upon them. You can feel sensations in these parts, such as heat or cold, and you will know if the area is tense or relaxed. You will feel their size and shape and also know that it is possible you haven't thought about your elbow or your big toe in such a focused way in years!

The Unconscious Mind

This is the right brain and its activities are out of your conscious awareness. For instance, it regulates your heartbeat, breathing, hormones and digestion without you even knowing about it. It looks after your elbow and big toe without you having to focus on them for their health and functioning.

Have you ever been travelling with your head in a book or a paper and find yourself unaware of how much time or many stations have passed? Have you ever driven from A to B and had no recollection of what happened on the way? This is when you are in a more unconscious mind state, where there is no time and where activities can happen without your conscious mind being there – and they still happen.

When you learnt a complex physical skill, like cycling, driving or operating machinery, remember how you did one thing at a time, concentrating really hard, and then added something else like steering, changing gear or changing the speed of the equipment? We can all remember when we learnt something and how hard it seemed to get all the elements in a row. Once learnt, it goes from conscious activity where you know and are thinking about everything, to unconscious activity where you just do it without even knowing you are doing it. This is how the unconscious mind operates; you are not aware of its vast power and how much it does for you.

The right brain is also where all your experiences, memories and knowledge are stored. They are stored in visual form together with the feelings and senses (touch, sight, sound, smell, taste, emotions). There is a view that when you sleep, this is the time information from the day is passed from your conscious into the storage that is your unconscious, from your short-term memory to your long-term memory.

The unconscious mind does not function with words. It also has no concept of time, or past, present or future. Everything is now. The unconscious mind does not have the analytical skills of the conscious, so everything in the unconscious is real. It cannot make a distinction between what you have imagined and what is actually real. It is not judgemental; it is creative, artistic, random, and its job is to move you towards your goals or ambitions.

UNDERSTANDING YOUR RIGHT BRAIN

It is important to understand the functioning of the unconscious as it is the side of the mind that protects us and allows us to function. As it is not analytical, however, it can sometimes do things for us that we may not consciously require. Take as an example the scenario of going for your first driving test. You have been imagining it in your mind – how nervous you are, how you will fluff your three-point turn. Your Inner Dialogue is 'I'm going to fail, I'm useless at driving' etc. What you have given the unconscious is memory of how you have failed. When you go to your test, your unconscious searches through its memory to see what it know about driving tests. So the result will be that it recalls nervousness, fluffing the three-point turn and failing. This is what Slim by Suggestion calls an 'unconscious programme' – stored information which will kick into operation when you stimulate the recall of anything real or imagined that you have done or thought about. It is exactly the same with the information you have stored about weight and what happens when you diet.

TEN EASY STEPS — STEP 1

If the associations in your mind about diets or dieting include misery, guilt, deprivation and failure, then you can expect more of the same if you start another diet. So Step 1 is for you to begin to overwrite the old programme with fresh, new information – this time you are going on a healthy eating programme, and your Inner Dialogue, as mentioned in Chapter 2, will be reinforcing this new vocabulary. As far as you can, just delete the word diets/dieting from your mind – don't let them be part of your Inner Dialogue and don't use the words in speech. Your CD tracks will reinforce this new information about healthy eating and being successful and motivated directly to your unconscious mind to give you a blueprint in your imagination that is accepted as true, and therefore must be delivered to you in actuality.

WHY WE USE SELF-HYPNOSIS

Listening to the CD will allow you to access a different brain-wave frequency which allows easier access to the unconscious. It will allow you to create new information that will be supportive to your goals on the programme.

There are four brain-wave frequencies as measured by an electro-encephalograph: alpha, beta, delta and theta:

Beta – Waking State
This is the frequency we are in during our waking hours. It is the frequency of conscious activity, involving rational, logical thinking and doing. The brain is functioning at its most rapid, dealing with information and activity.

Alpha – Half-awake State
The Alpha state is when we are deeply relaxed. You can recognize this brain-wave activity as that level of relaxation just before you go to sleep or just before you wake up. It is like a day-dream state, and it is when you

access the unconscious part of your mind. During this frequency and the Theta frequency is the ideal time to make use of the imagination to create new programmes in the unconscious as the brain-wave activity is conducive to accepting suggestions. This is the brain-wave activity you will access when you are in self-hypnosis listening to the CD tracks. The physical feeling will be of heavy limbs or deep relaxation; mentally, it can be a feeling of drifting away into your own inner world. It is ideal to sit or lie down in a warm place as your body temperature can drop a few degrees. Sometimes people hear the words on the CD and sometimes they don't; it really doesn't matter how you experience it as the unconscious mind can hear everything. By using the Alpha state, you can give new information to your unconscious to create changes and to deprogramme and reprogramme yourself with new and positive information and so develop new behaviours.

Children between 7 and 14 years of age function predominately in this half-waking state and are very receptive to suggestions from all sources. They need to be highly suggestible in order to learn and to store information quickly and easily.

Do not listen to the CD whilst driving or operating machinery.

Theta – Dreaming State

These brain waves occur when the brain is dreaming while you are asleep or in deep relaxation, and you may not be aware of your body. Much information is stored by the unconscious during this frequency. When you listen to your CD, you will fluctuate between Alpha and Theta.

Children under the age of seven predominantly use this frequency, and it is the most highly suggestible brain-wave pattern. Children up to this age have to learn and absorb so much information, and this frequency allows rapid and direct storage of that knowledge.

Delta – Deep Sleep State

This frequency occurs in deep sleep, while under anaesthetic or unconscious, when the brain is functioning very slowly.

Why Reprogramming the Unconscious is so Important

- Anything you imagine is accepted as real and true in your unconscious mind.
- Your behaviour and emotions follow what the unconscious mind has stored about that situation.
- If you try to use willpower, your conscious wishes from your conscious mind, and this is not in line with the blueprint or programme that is stored with the related information in your unconscious mind, you will fail. The unconscious mind, by using Inner Dialogue, emotions and behaviours, will override your conscious wishes. When willpower and imagination are in conflict, the imagination will always win. You are likely to feel highly emotional.
- If you have always failed in your attempts to lose excess body fat, then that is what is stored as information. Your next 'diet' may start off successfully, but then you will find yourself doing things and experiencing a turmoil of emotions which are not in line with your wish to lose excess body fat. This turmoil and being unable to resist out-of-control eating is the sign that your conscious wishes and your unconscious mind are not working together. You can experience urges, compulsions, bizarre behaviour and feel as if you are caught in the middle of a battle between the left and right sides of the brain. Your unconscious will impel you to fail as that is what it knows; that is what has happened before. The unconscious is programmed to keep you where you are

(or worse) because it believes that that is your aim, your goal. So willpower won't work.

- Using the unconscious mind by giving it the positive outcomes of your Slim by Suggestion activities through the CD tracks is a key way for you to move forward and make changes.

Negative Thinking and Excuses

The mind will provide another type of dialogue to prevent you from moving towards change – this we call negative thinking and it can work very well, in conjunction with your Inner Critic, to stop you making any changes. This type of thinking supports the current unconscious mind programming and it is very, very unhelpful to the process of reprogramming your unconscious.

Have you ever been somewhere where it was cold then, when you go somewhere similar, you are cold before you get through the door? Experience tells me 'big houses are cold' so my body manifests the physical reaction to ward off cold before I experience actual cold.

Places of worship have many associations. Depending on their nature, they will, if allowed, affect your next experience of them. If, for example, your mind associates churches with a happy occasion, all the cross-references you will get from your mind before you go to a church will be happy. The mind, however, is better at providing you with negative reminders. The most important part of its job is to protect you against emotional or physical hurt, so it is set up to give you recall of unpleasant things before it will get anything pleasant out of the memory stores! Prevention of pain or harm is the most important task; pleasure takes second place.

Using the church analogy, you will remember first the funeral, then the four weddings – your mind warns you by supplying a constant stream of 'last time it was unpleasant, last time you felt afraid, last time you got really hurt', to protect you from harm. This protective form of thinking constitutes much of what is called 'negative thinking'. It is your own thinking and can be totally under your control once you understand your internal thought processes and the principles behind them.

As well as physical protection, everyone acquires ways over time of defending themselves against emotional pain. Many of these defences and protective responses (defence mechanisms) are developed when we are young, inexperienced and immature. We may invent our own defences, but we also copy behaviour from any role models that are handy, like parents, peers or other significant adults. It is essential to understand that once we have acquired and perfected a defence reaction it becomes incorporated unconsciously so that we think it is part of our nature. These reactions are activated automatically every time a situation is presented. The mind will search until it finds matching or corresponding information or associated experiences. It will not only find the pictures and images of associated events but it will locate *associated emotions, previous behaviour,* physical sensations and thoughts around that event.

Because the defence reactions are automatically activated, we will then experience the way we are thinking as an essential part of our make-up, as if it is normal and a part of our personality. We also believe that our behaviours and automatic responses are a part of the way we are:

- 'That's the way I am and there's nothing I can do about it.'
- 'I know myself, and there's nothing that can help me.'
- 'I get no help, and there's nothing I can do.'
- 'I'm never lucky; there's always a misfortune waiting to happen.'

About Your Brain

- 'It's my nature to be emotional.'
- 'I'm sensitive, and that's why I get so stressed out.'
- 'It's too late now to change.'
- 'It's just not fair; why do I have a weight problem?'

Excuses like these are common internally-held defensive beliefs. They stop you moving forward into new territory – just because your mind believes, from previous experience or learning, that it may be dangerous. It might be dangerous, but then again, it might not. Your mind does not know the answer; the mind does not know the outcome of a future event; only experience will find out.

Another reason why these automatic defensive reactions are holding you back is that the unconscious will manifest for you what you consciously or unconsciously believe to be true. It will see the excuses as your goal, the direction you require, and move towards it. So if you think 'Change is too difficult', then change will be made too difficult.

Joan's Story

Joan had inexplicable cravings for food, and binged regularly. She would open a packet of biscuits and find herself halfway through the second pack before she 'knew what was happening'.

Through her Healthy-living Diary (*Chapter 7*), we examined what was going on when she experienced her cravings – what she was doing, whom she was with, the time of day, how she was feeling, etc. When we discussed it, Joan pointed out that there was a connection, but she couldn't figure it out. The connection was that the bingeing happened on evenings when it was her turn to pick up her small daughter (aged four) and friends on the nursery run.

When we talked through the situation, we discovered that Joan felt very uneasy and tense as soon as she walked into the nursery school premises. She began to consider her background and remembered that her mother had described her as being very clingy when she went to nursery. The penny began to drop for Joan … even though she'd had a great and enjoyable time at primary and secondary school, her experience of nursery was frightening.

Her food cravings and bingeing were her behaviour in response to the emotion of fear, first experienced at nursery when she was four. Joan had not consciously recalled anything about nursery at all.

Sarah's Story

Sarah had been overweight since she was a child. She was a highly capable person and she and her family couldn't understand why she was unable to lose weight. One theory was that her weight was in her genetic make-up. But what was actually happening to Sarah was that, in her unconscious mind, she truly believed she was and had always been fat. So whenever Sarah decided to go on a diet, her conscious mind scanned her unconscious mind and failed to find an example of dieting successfully. So Sarah lost a few pounds, maybe even a few stone, but because this did not make sense in her unconscious mind, the weight went back on. Sarah had no unconscious picture of what being slim was; her mind told her that she was overweight and always had been.

Kate's Story

Kate's weight had fluctuated since she was a teenager. She was totally frustrated and just couldn't understand where her motivation had gone. She decided to contact a Slim by Suggestion therapist. During a discussion, Kate said that she would really like to lose weight so that she could start to enjoy life, the way slim people did. She said that she would like to be nine stone. She was asked when was the last time she was nine stone. Her reply was five years ago. The therapist then asked Kate what she did five years ago in order to get to nine stone. Kate said that her marriage broke up and that she had no desire to eat during that difficult time.

What was really going on here was that Kate's unconscious mind had made the connection that being nine stone brings emotional turmoil, rejection and hurt, even though consciously she had not made the connection. Her mental picture was connecting nine stone with emotional pain. We all have this protective mechanism that defends us from unnecessary emotional trauma. Therefore, Kate unconsciously stops herself returning to this emotional state. Until Kate breaks the unconscious connection, she will find it very difficult to lose weight and even harder to maintain it at nine stone.

The example of Kate and the others are just some from hundreds with similar themes. Unconsciously, there is always a valid, and usually protective, reason to stay overweight, even when consciously you desire to be slim.

In the past, you have probably spent most of your time thinking about your weight, about how much you want to reduce your weight, let go of excess fat etc. By doing this, you are reinforcing and manifesting the very things you do not want!

Remember, the more you see, think and talk to yourself about how overweight you are, the more you can guarantee your unconscious mind will think this is what you want.

So we are going to encourage your unconscious mind to develop inner tools to combat this negative programming by utilizing our techniques. Together we can start to release negative programming very easily without any great conscious effort to generate a stronger internal mechanism to achieve your goal. Your unconscious mind, or control centre, is real and alert and can be reprogrammed so that you can achieve your goals.

SOME THINGS TO TRY

When you consider your negative thinking or the excuses you give yourself, check them out to see if they are old defence mechanisms. These mechanisms also love to use 'out-of-control' eating as part of the defensive package. Even if an excuse or thought pattern is not an old defence, check it out and see if it is relevant to you today.

In order to get in control of your eating, you need to prepare for forthcoming events or experiences which may or may not already have some triggers stored in your unconscious.

Money
Too much money or not enough? There are many fears around money, often linked to concepts of materialism or aspirations, success and failure. For men, particularly strong beliefs concern the ability to provide. Keeping up with the Joneses.

- What happens to your thinking and behaviour if you have to host a dinner party for your partner's seriously wealthy boss? Or go to a dinner party at a special venue?

Alcohol

Not only your own consumption (which can be a binge in itself) but that of others.

- How does it affect you when you see your partner, friends, colleagues, complete strangers, drinking or drunk, or teetotal?

Relationships

Using someone else as an excuse for not losing weight is another way of avoiding your own emotions and behaviour. No one else is responsible for your excess body fat. You are.

- 'My parents expect us all to sit down together for a full three-course meal.'

The Situation is Hopeless

In life, events occur that are not always in your control. You may want to be able to control events, but it will not always be possible, and the outcome may not be predictable. All or nothing thinking is defensive (yet not constructive).

- 'I'll never be able to get this done in time.'
- 'It's impossible.'
- 'I'll never be able to lose body fat.'

Taking on Other People's Problems

As excuses go, this one is sophisticated – an individual will take on other people's problems in order to avoid their own emotions. It is rather like creating a vacuum in which to suck everything and everyone up in order to avoid your own issues and thoughts.

This is also highly stressful because you actually take on someone else's problems and issues to worry about, in an attempt to avoid your own, and they may have problems worse than your own!

- Watch out for people around trying to 'help'. They are being needy and dependent as they want your problems in order to avoid their own.
- 'I can't do my Emotional Journal today because I promised X that I would do their shopping.'
- 'I've got to go out with Janet today as she is so upset. Unfortunately, she has chosen a bistro and that means wine (sugar), more wine (sugar) and fatty food (pizza).'

Being a Born Worrier

Habitual worriers are created, not born. It is a habit to thrive on worrying about everyone and everything. If you ask your mind for negative and defensive thoughts, it is its job to supply you with suitably negative answers. If you ask your mind for positive and creative thoughts, which are equally protective, it will supply you with positive and creative thoughts. It does not matter to the mind; it only responds to what you demand.

- Try it. Stop negative worrying thinking and choose positive thoughts instead. It will make no difference to any outcomes, and make you happier and well-balanced, more in control of your own thinking. **You choose the thoughts you think**.
- Consider what is going on in your head – are you giving yourself the wrong messages, are you misleading your mind into thinking the wrong sort of goals?

Whenever you make an excuse to yourself – check it out, then chuck it out.

6

About You

This chapter contains questionnaires designed to give you an opportunity to assess where you are at this minute in your emotional world. Slim by Suggestion is a holistic or 'whole-person' programme, so the questionnaires look at your living habits, emotional life, stress, beliefs, motivation and personality traits. Their aim is to give you a guide to yourself. Consider this as a starting point for the programme. It's not an ordeal!

The questionnaires that follow are for you only, and for the answers to be valid and helpful to you, please answer all the questions spontaneously and truthfully. What we mean is that, when you read the question, just put in the first answer that comes to mind. This is likely to be your real self talking, not the voice of your Inner Critic or its cohorts.

There are no right or wrong answers; the purpose of the questionnaires is to help you understand your internal dynamics. This is your 'before' stage of the programme and there is an evaluation for you to look at which will offer indications as to your weaknesses and your strengths. After your eight weeks on the Slim by Suggestion programme, you can redo the questionnaires to help you measure your progress. Record your answers on a separate sheet of paper, or photocopy the questionnaires, so when you come to redo the questionnaires at the end of the programme, you read the questions without the influence of the previous results.

Sometimes it is too easy to focus just on weight loss (removal of excess body fat) and to ignore, or not consider, some of the other aspects of behaviour and self-worth which need to change when you are working on your whole self. These include your self-image, your physical and mental self.

Eating Evaluation

Read each question and tick the YES box if the statement is true for you. Tick the NO box if the statement does not apply to you. Answer as truthfully and spontaneously as you can. If in doubt – if the question sometimes applies and sometimes does not – tick both boxes.

	YES	NO
Do you eat when you are disappointed with someone or something?		
Is eating an important source of pleasure in your life?		
Do you have a tendency to eat when you are disappointed with your own behaviour?		
Do you sometimes hide what you eat from others?		
Are you more than 20 per cent over your ideal weight?		
Do you sometimes have uncontrollable food cravings?		
When you are on a diet do you feel deprived and/or impatient?		
Are you/have you been obsessed by the scales?		
In some ways, do you dread reaching your ideal weight?		

	YES	NO
Is food a big issue in your life?		
When you wake in the morning, do you think about what you can eat during the day?		
Are you aware of your hunger levels i.e. very hungry, not very hungry, full up?		
Are you afraid to bring home some foods?		
Do you eat just because others are eating?		

Now move on to the next section.

How Do You Eat?

Read the statements below. The ones you agree with, tick YES/TRUE. The ones you disagree with, tick NO/FALSE.

	YES TRUE	NO FALSE
Eating is enjoyable, but it doesn't rule me.		
I usually wait until I'm hungry to eat.		
I feel comfortable with the way I look.		
I never eat when I'm standing in front of the refrigerator with the door open.		
I feel normal about the way that I eat.		

	YES TRUE	NO FALSE
I know how to plan my eating for social events so that I don't go overboard.		
I can go to a party and not be focused on the food and how much I can eat.		
I can go away for the weekend and feel comfortable that I won't gain weight.		
I know exactly how much I eat every day.		
I know what foods I enjoy more than others.		
I am honest with myself about what I eat.		
I can keep to a diet where they tell you exactly what to eat.		
I will stop short of finishing my food and clearing my plate if it means I will feel too full.		
I only eat food that I really feel like eating.		
I rarely eat something straight from the container, tin or packet.		
I don't need to hide my food.		
I don't need to hide my shopping.		
I never feel guilty after I've eaten.		
I can go to a buffet dinner and leave without feeling stuffed.		
I have a good idea how much I eat and drink every day.		
I don't feel depressed about my weight.		
I never feel hopeless about the way I eat or how much I weigh.		
I don't feel caught up in the dieting/bingeing cycle.		

About You

	YES TRUE	NO FALSE
I never eat off others' plates when I'm clearing the table.		
I don't pick at leftovers.		
I take good care of myself by eating foods I enjoy and those that are good for me.		
I know what constitutes healthy eating.		

Score two points for each answer to Yes/True _____

Score no points for each answer to No/False _____

Your Self-image

Rate each of your answers to the following statements as follows:

0 = Totally Disagree

1 = Could disagree

2 = Could agree

3 = Completely agree

SELF-IMAGE – SECTION 1	0	1	2	3
My life is on hold. I'm not getting anywhere. It's as if I'm stuck.				
Everybody thinks I'm all right, but I know I'm not.				
I don't involve myself in activities, particularly if I don't know that I will be successful.				
I am quick to criticize other people, to their face verbally or in my own mind.				

SELF-IMAGE – SECTION 1 *cont.*	0	1	2	3
I am a do-gooder. I support the underdog.				
When things don't go well it is often down to me, my fault.				
People cannot be trusted.				
I find it hard to make friends.				
I feel inferior to other people.				
I'm a sensitive person.				
I'm concerned about what other people think of me.				
I have to prove that I am the best at whatever I attempt.				
Successful people are often selfish and walk over other people's feelings.				
I rarely do anything right.				
SELF-IMAGE – SECTION 2				
I can get angry over the slightest thing.				
People have a tendency to be really irritating.				
I can be very heavy-handed and sometimes I can break things.				
I can be snappy.				
I often lash out verbally if I think I'm being picked on.				
It's better to get your point across before others do.				
I prefer it when I'm in charge.				
I criticize others (particularly if I think they're going to criticize me).				
I don't get on with people who are intolerant.				

69

SELF-IMAGE – SECTION 3	0	1	2	3
People have a tendency to ignore my viewpoint.				
I don't bother to put my opinion across.				
There are times when I feel I just can't be bothered.				
People can be very fickle.				
I don't like to draw attention to myself.				
It is often easier to get what you want by being underhand/devious.				
I spend a lot of time concerned with what will happen in the future.				
It is easy for me to think of the negative viewpoint.				
I won't try anything new because it might not work out or I might make a show of myself.				

Add up your score for Section 1 _____

Add up your score for Section 2 _____

Add up your score for Section 3 _____ and continue the questionnaire.

Personality Traits

Personality traits can influence our attitudes and behaviour. On the questionnaire below, circle the number on the scale that best characterizes your behaviour for each trait. The higher the number, the stronger you consider this trait. For instance, if you are not competitive, then your answer is number 1; if you are very competitive, your answer is 8; if you are somewhere in between, circle the number which best represents you.

Casual about meetings or appointments.	1 2 3 4 5 6 7 8	Never late.
Not competitive.	1 2 3 4 5 6 7 8	Very competitive.
Never feel rushed, even under pressure.	1 2 3 4 5 6 7 8	Always rushed.
Take things one at a time.	1 2 3 4 5 6 7 8	Try to do many things at once; think about what I am going to do next.
Slow doing things, measured activity.	1 2 3 4 5 6 7 8	Fast eating, walking, talking, movements etc.
Express feelings.	1 2 3 4 5 6 7 8	Sit on feelings, squash feelings down.
Many interests.	1 2 3 4 5 6 7 8	Few interests outside work.

Add up your score and multiply the answer by 3. _____ × 3 = _____
Continue the questionnaire.

Emotional Assessment

Stress and emotions are two distinct things – they can operate individually in a person but often they are interlinked. For instance, a stressful situation may trigger emotions such as guilt, anger and frustration. In the same way, feeling some types of emotion, such as fear, hostility and aggressiveness, can trigger stress symptoms like sweating, racing heart, tight stomach and clenched jaw.

Rate each of your answers to the following statements:

	0	1	2	3
I try and help other people with their problems. 0=Never 1=Sometimes 2=Often 3=Usually				
I find other people very demanding. 0=Never 1=Sometimes 2=Quite often 3=Very often				
I am happy in my own company. 0=Always 1=Sometimes 2=Not very happy 3=Unhappy				
I expect myself to do well at whatever I try. 0=Not true 1=Sometimes true 2=Often true 3=Always true				
I have no one to confide in. 0=Disagree 1=Sometimes disagree 2=Sometimes agree 3=Totally agree				
My life consists of going to work and sleeping. 0=Completely disagree 1=Sometimes disagree 2=Sometimes agree 3=Totally agree				
When I need to change, I find it easy as I can be adaptable. 0=Completely disagree 1=Sometimes disagree 2=Sometimes agree 3=Totally agree				
There is a saying: 'There is a time and a place for everything', and this is true. 0=Completely disagree 1=Sometimes disagree 2=Sometimes agree 3=Totally agree				
If I think that someone doesn't like me I get very upset. 0=Not at all 1=Not really bothered 2=A little bit upset 3=Very upset				
When there is a problem I always look at it from the positive viewpoint. 0=Always 1=Usually 2=Sometimes 3=Never				
I don't care about anything or anybody. 0=Never 1=Sometimes 2=Quite often 3=Very often				

	0	1	2	3
I don't seem to have enough time to get things done. 0=Untrue 1=Sometimes run out of time 2=Mostly run out of time 3=Never have enough time				
People are not able to change after 35; they are set in their ways. 0=Completely disagree 1=Sometimes disagree 2=Sometimes agree 3=Totally agree				
I can be upset by the smallest incident. 0=Never 1=Sometimes 2= Quite often 3=Most of the time				
I feel like my world is just about to come crashing down around me. 0=Never 1=Sometimes 2=Quite often 3=Most of the time				
People tell me I'm over-sensitive. 0=Completely disagree 1=Sometimes disagree 2=Sometimes agree 3=Totally agree				
I try to treat others as I would like to be treated myself – but other people disappoint me. 0=Totally untrue 1=Sometimes true: 2=Often true: 3=Totally true				
When I make a mistake, I forget about it immediately. 0=Always 1=Usually 2=Yes, but it's not easy 3=I'm unable to forget my mistake				
People have told me I am a perfectionist. 0=Totally untrue 1=Sometimes true 2=Often true 3=totally true				
Deep down I think life is unfair. 0=Totally untrue 1=Sometimes true 2=Often True 3=Totally True				

Add up your score _____

Continue with the questionnaire.

Stress Assessment

Here is a list of stress-related symptoms. Please rate each of them on the following scale which will indicate how often you have experienced them, if at all, during the last 21 days (exclude any symptoms that are the result of exercise or menopause).

    0 = Not at all

    1 = Occasionally

    2 = Often

    3 = Most of the time

	0	1	2	3
Palpitations (heart seems loud and fast/seems to skip a beat).				
Breathlessness/rapid breathing.				
Chest pains or discomfort.				
Pain/discomfort in shoulder, neck and/or back.				
Dizziness or feeling unsteady.				
Tingling or numbness.				
Ringing or buzzing in the ears.				
Hot and/or cold flushes.				
Tension in jaw, neck and/or facial muscles.				
Sweating.				
Skin irritation or susceptibility to allergies.				
Lapses in memory.				
Feeling of nausea/sickness.				
Waking in the early hours.				

	0	1	2	3
Difficulty getting back to sleep/difficulty sleeping.				
Suffer from upset stomach/diarrhoea.				
Bladder needs to be emptied a lot.				
Can't settle down to get on with things – procrastination.				
Headaches/migraines.				
Difficulty in concentration.				
Dry mouth and/or difficulty in swallowing.				
Stomach feels knotted.				
Head like cotton wool/thinking in a fog.				
Legs twitch in bed.				
Feelings of unreality/detachment.				
Near to tears.				
Low energy level.				
Worrying (for instance, a particular thought won't go away).				
Irritability or restlessness.				
Drinking too much alcohol.				
Eating habits out of control.				
Feelings of inadequacy.				
Moodiness.				
Temper outbursts or aggressive incidents.				
Hyperactivity.				
Inability to relax.				

Add up your score _____

About You

Now move on to the Personal Assessment section to discover what your personal score means at this time.

Personal Assessment

You will have marked your score on your separate sheets of paper or photocopied completed questionnaires. Use the guide below to help you understand what the questionnaires reveal. There are no right or wrong scores. The questionnaires are designed to give you some information about yourself which you can use to make positive changes to your mental, emotional and physical weight.

EATING EVALUATION

If you answered YES to any of the questions, then you are not eating when you are hungry; you are eating for other reasons. Some of the reasons you may be aware of; others may be unconsciously-held beliefs or habitual behaviour due to an unconscious programme operating in your mind. What the evaluation does reveal is that for every YES answer, there is a difference of opinion between your conscious desires and your actual behaviour around food. It is really important to look at all your answers (without the help and assistance of The Inner Critic, The Pleaser and The Perfectionist) and think about how they affect your eating patterns. You are likely to find that these powerful unconscious programmes in your mind are some of the root causes of the compulsions, emotional turmoil and blocks which are part of 'out-of-control' eating.

HOW DO YOU EAT?

Consider the individual questions to which you have answered NO/FALSE.
Each of these scenarios shows where you need to change how you behave
in order to achieve your goal of being slimmer, healthier and in control of
your eating. For instance, if you answered FALSE to the question ' I rarely
eat something from the container, tin or packet', we can assume that you
do eat straight from the packet, tin or container. This may be undesirable
behaviour if you want to stay in control of what you are consuming. Many
people have found that if they take the strategy of putting out two or three
items on a plate, sitting down and enjoying the occasion with no
distractions, they can savour the food, chew slowly and feel fuller. This
prevents the 'guilt and lying syndrome': 'Oops, I've just finished the whole
packet ... well, there were only a few in there; it won't harm my healthy-
eating programme!' You may like to reflect in your Emotional Journal (*see
next chapter*) about those unwanted behaviours you have discovered, and
consider what you can do to behave in a different way.

Looking at the score that you have recorded:
All the FALSE/NO answers you have ticked give you an area in your
emotional or behavioural life that you can start to work on. If you answered
TRUE/YES to the statement 'I feel comfortable about the way I look', then
this is a positive thought showing emotional balance that you can use to
encourage yourself, even when you know you have answered FALSE/NO
to the statement 'I never feel guilty after I have eaten'. If you do feel guilty
after eating, this shows the opposite – an emotional imbalance you need to
work on. Some of the FALSE/NO questions are concerned with behaviour
you will want to change and gain control over, and some are to do with

identifying particular scenarios when you are unable to consume normally. For instance, if you go to a buffet and lose control, or gain weight when you take a weekend break, you know there are pressures around those events that you don't respond to in the way you would like.

A score of less than 28:
You can acknowledge that there are some significant blockages and unwanted programmes at an unconscious level that the Slim by Suggestion programme is designed to help you overcome. Remember who is in charge – *you* – not the inner voices who are likely to be strong if you have this type of score. You are doing something positive for yourself by taking the easy steps of the programme.

A score between 30 and 46:
You need to look at your behaviour in detail and start to work on some of the contributory compulsions, blocks or emotional turmoil that surround this behaviour. In addition, you are likely to have a poor body image and low self-esteem, which you need to build through the CD and this programme. You are moving in the direction that will lead you to being in control of your eating/drinking as your unconscious comes into line with your conscious desires.

A score between 48 and 54:
Your self-esteem is high and there is a balance between your emotions and your behaviour. You can congratulate yourself that you are able to make unconscious shifts and act upon them to give you the behaviour you consciously desire.

SELF-IMAGE QUESTIONNAIRES

Your answers to these questionnaires can help you gauge more about your personality type. This can play an important role in relation to how you eat and drink and whether or not your consumption is triggered by factors other than hunger.

Section 1
A score between 0 and 9:

Your self-esteem is high and you are emotionally well balanced. Your relationships with people are excellent and you are able to choose, consciously, what it is you want, without any old, unconsciously-held beliefs or blocks causing you emotional turmoil. You are self-confident with a good body image. You naturally spend time on yourself to keep your confidence and motivation levels high.

A score between 10 and 14:

You are confident with good self-esteem. Most of your relationships are satisfactory and you are mainly happy in your life. Your level of self-esteem may become dented with the ups and downs of ordinary life, so we recommend you use your CD and emotional journal to work through anything that makes you feel any loss of motivation, or negativity. Make sure you do everything you can to keep life stimulating and your mental faculties sharp. Guard against the tendencies of your Perfectionist and/or Pleaser.

A score between 15 and 22:

Your self-esteem levels could be higher, together with your body image and confidence. Use all the techniques available through the 10 easy steps of Slim by Suggestion to boost your self-image and confidence and to re-evaluate any beliefs which may be self-limiting and cause blocks and emotional turmoil. Consistently negotiate with and turn down your Inner Dialogue as The Inner Critic, Perfectionist and Pleaser are holding you back from positive and self-supporting Internal Dialogue.

A score of 23 or more:
Your confidence and self-esteem levels need considerable improvement for you to feel you can have a good relationship with yourself. Your relationships and self-beliefs are in need of an overhaul. With consistent use of the techniques in this programme and the CD tracks, you can make good progress. Your Inner Critic, Perfectionist and Pleaser parts are too influential upon you and are holding you back. Make sure that you continue to be motivated to follow the 10 steps of the Slim by Suggestion programme – a lack of motivation will be due to the self-limiting beliefs, emotional and behavioural habits which need to change in line with your conscious wishes. Take small, consistent steps towards your goal every day and be sure to congratulate yourself for all the good things you do.

Section 2
A score between 0 and 9:
No one could describe you as aggressive. You can observe the actions and activities of others without getting involved or reacting. Alternatively, you may be not very in touch with your feelings and you may keep the world at a distance. Re-evaluate your score at the end of the Slim by Suggestion programme.

A score between 10 and 17:
Your level of aggression can be described as average. You just need to ensure that the aggression or any aggressive reaction is used for positive and motivating activity and to achieve the goals you want. Be on your

guard if you sense a greater level of aggression or reactions, as you may be tempted to push these feelings down with food or drink. Use all of the techniques and information on the programme to keep you in touch with your feelings and sustain your level of self-esteem.

A score between 18 and 27:
You may find that experiencing this high level of aggression is not making life comfortable for you. The aggressive energy may be misdirected onto others or you may internalize it against yourself. Either way, it is not helping you feel emotionally in control or supporting a good level of self-esteem. Try from now to redirect this aggressive energy towards positive goals and your own self-improvement. Use all the techniques and information on the programme and bear this level of aggression in mind when you are using your Emotional Journal (*see next chapter*). Try to look for patterns relating to aggressive or unpleasant interactions and how you eat and drink; there may be a link as you use food to push down unpleasant feelings and thoughts. Work on you and turn down the volume of your Inner Critic.

Section 3

A score between 0 and 9:
You could be described as passive or you could be aggressive. Or you may not be in touch with your feelings and you may keep the world at a distance. Re-evaluate your score at the end of the Slim by Suggestion programme. Consider how you answered the questions. You could use your Emotional Journal (*see next chapter*) to discuss some of the questions and their implications about your level of passivity, interaction or confidence.

A score between 10 and 17:

You have an average level of passivity, and you might like to think about the more passive side of your personality and how it affects your life. There is a tendency for you to avoid taking full control, and your Pleaser and Inner Critic, together with your Perfectionist, may conspire to keep you standing still. Doing nothing is the most protective activity to avoid risk. This tendency may urge you to quit the programme – this is a learnt behaviour and part of unconscious self-limiting beliefs. Use all the techniques and information on the programme to keep you in touch with your feelings and sustain your level of self-esteem.

A score between 18 and 27:

You can be described as very passive. This means that, at the very least, you are not being true to yourself. Your Inner Critic is likely to be with you every waking moment, and your Pleaser will not let you rest. It is important for you to work on negotiating with all the parts of your Inner Dialogue on an ongoing basis. You need to make a commitment to yourself that you are going to take small, consistent steps towards your objectives. Use all the techniques and the CD track and do something every day towards the 10 easy steps of the programme. You will soon see benefits.

These Self-image Questionnaires may reveal that you have a mixed personality – partly passive and partly aggressive. This is a very common combination and suggests that you need to recognize your strengths and weaknesses when you put all your techniques into use. If you have scored very passive and very aggressive, start to look at with whom, what and where these behaviours and thinking occur, and consider how the emotional fallout impacts on your pattern of eating and drinking.

For moderate scores, consider what gains you receive from behaving passively or aggressively.

PERSONALITY TRAITS

This questionnaire looks at whether you are a Type A or a Type B personality. This A/B personality description is a common measure used in many psychometric assessments.

21–90	B Type
90–99	B+ Type
100–105	A– Type
106–119	A Type
120 or more	A+ Type

Type A Personalities

If you are any of the A Types, you need to be aware that this reflects thought patterns and Inner Dialogue which lead to certain behaviours and emotional turmoil. These, in turn, may have a significant impact on your level of stress.

A Types typically undertake more than one job at a time, and never feel they have enough time. They make very good employees as they will do anything to get the job done. They are the type who will not use all their holiday allowance; they'll come to work early and leave later than anyone else. They may try to cram too much work into a given time, resulting in a race against the clock and considerable pressure. They do most things at 100 miles per hour.

If you are a Type A personality, it is a good indication that you have a tendency to be competitive about almost everything. Your natural reactions to situations and events may include hostility and aggression. You will have a big Perfectionist part. You tend to take on more than your share of responsibility and may not be very good at delegating.

In addition, Type A personalities may be very ambitious to achieve their personal goals. These may be poorly selected and create unconscious confusion and compulsions. A Types can have high levels of mental activity, and some may be hyperactive.

Type B Personalities

B Types need to guard against complacency and prevarication. They can feel very stuck, hopeless and helpless, and they may show signs of stress when they are too slow off the mark or cannot seem to get things done. Type B personalities are more able to relax and enjoy life than A Types, and they are less likely to be materialistic and work-orientated. B Types have the ability to be in control over their thinking, which will lead them to deal with events as they happen, difficulties as they occur and relationships in a calm way.

It's important to realize that it is your thinking that determines the stress reactions you have. Type A people will need to try to take on more of the opposite B traits, and consider their attitudes to delegation, time-management, assertiveness, relaxation and goal-setting. Type B personalities will need to take on more of the positive traits of the Type A. The most highly successful people have the best parts of both.

EMOTIONAL ASSESSMENT

A score between 0 and 5:

With this score, it is likely that you have not answered the questionnaire fully, or you may not be in touch with your feelings. You may like to keep the world at a distance. Re-evaluate your score at the end of the Slim by Suggestion programme.

A score between 6 and 10:

This demonstrates that you are well-balanced emotionally.

A score between 11 and 14:

This is an average score. You are likely to be in control of your emotions and feel well-balanced most of the time. There may be some particular circumstances, situations or people that trigger your emotions, and you may react with out-of-control eating and/or drinking. Use all 10 steps of the programme to find out which situations cause your emotions to be triggered – there will be underlying beliefs or unconscious blockages for you to work on.

A score between 16 and 25:

You are more than averagely emotional. As a result, you are over-sensitive about certain situations/events/people. The easy steps of the programme will begin to benefit you very shortly as you start to recognize and work on your emotions and their triggers. Start to treat yourself better by ensuring that your Inner Critic and Pleaser parts are in your control, not in control. Give yourself plenty of support and positive thoughts.

A score of 26 or more:

You are very emotional. This may make your life feel like a roller-coaster ride, and you want to get off. Being as emotional or sensitive as you are is not all negative and damaging. There are many positive sides to being an emotional person as you are able to experience the highs more intensely too. However, many of your out-of-control feelings around food may be due to your emotional make-up. You will need to recognize the emotional triggers and the underlying beliefs creating turmoil and work on them with the steps of the programme. Listen to your CD as much as possible; get off to a strong start. Start to consider yourself and treat yourself as you would like to be treated. Make sure that your Inner Critic and Pleaser parts are in your control, not in control. Give yourself plenty of support and positive thoughts.

STRESS ASSESSMENT

Stressed individuals have physical, emotional and behavioural symptoms. Your thinking processes and your Internal Dialogue in relation to situations and events cause you to respond in an emotional way and with a type of behaviour. You need to work on ways to break your patterns of thinking. It's really important to recognize your stress levels and then take a look at how your thinking produces the emotional and behavioural reactions. These behaviours can include the use of food and drink to push down the physiological side-effects of stress chemicals (adrenalin and cortisol). Prolonged and untreated stress can result in life-threatening illness and death. Stress can kill you.

A score between 0 and 9:
You may be out of touch with your body.

A score between 10 and 35:
This is well within the normal range. Recognize any changes in these symptoms to make sure that they do not increase in their intensity or frequency.

A score between 36 and 54:
We need a certain amount of stress. However, you will benefit from using the tools of the programme to help reduce the frequency of some of your symptoms. Stress chemicals lower the resistance of your immune system,

whose job it is to protect you from illness. This means that you are more susceptible to everyday infections like colds and flu. When under stress at this level, it is your weakest link that will cause you physical problems.

A score between 54 and 72:
You are experiencing harmful and unhealthy stress responses. When levels of the stress hormone cortisol stay raised for a long time, it can prevent certain acids being removed from our blood and this can cause stomach ulcers. Alongside this may come other physical ailments like headaches, muscle tension, bowel disorders, blood pressure, skin problems, asthma, and arthritis, multiple sclerosis, cancer and heart disease.

At this level of stress, your personality may become distorted as minor incidents cause you to blow a fuse, or over-react in some way. You are likely either to eat a lot less or eat even more, and you may be binge drinking. Your relationships with others are liable to come under pressure as you become over-critical or over-controlling.

Your emotional and behavioural responses are very all or nothing; you are either very energetic or feel like collapsing. The energy required by the body to cope with this long-term stress will have many physical and emotional effects. It is likely that your memory and ability to concentrate is much worse and anger and irritation are dangerously close to the top. Self-esteem is eroded and panic or despairing feelings are more and more frequent. Your thinking will be almost out of control and you may get into cycles of negative future worry, going over and over 'worst case scenarios'.

Start treating yourself better, NOW.

A score of 74 or more:
You are in serious danger of burnout. You can read the comments for the score above as well as this assessment. Every symptom you have scored as experiencing 'most of the time' is VERY unhealthy and damaging.

Burnout refers to feelings of extreme mental and physical exhaustion as a result of long-term stress. Your body is filled to the brim with stress biochemicals and your resources of energy are totally depleted. The effects on you are catastrophic as your reactions are sluggish and you find it hard to think straight. This level of stress is at the point where there is an inability to make decisions or cope with responsibility. Your ability to 'get the job done' will be seriously affected as your productivity is very low, motivation is low and inspiration non-existent. Your Perfectionist part is very strong and you may feel as if you don't even know yourself any more as your personality is suppressed. Fun people are serious; happy people are depressed; helpful people are careless; and life is hard.

You may need to rethink many things. A break or a holiday with no stress may be a first step. At the very least, you need to make changes. Look after yourself – use the easy steps of the programme and, in particular, use the CD at least twice a day consistently. Take change slowly with gradual exercise and a healthy-eating programme. You are at a low ebb; don't add more stress by attempting to achieve a miracle overnight.

Look out for patterns of thinking, emotional reactions and behaviour and work on them. Don't underestimate the seriousness of the damage you are doing to your body.

SOME THINGS TO THINK ABOUT

- Take some time to think about the information you have read about yourself. Please make sure that your Inner Critic is quiet and you are being supportive to yourself. The information from the questionnaires is an indicator about your strengths and weaknesses. Remember, nothing is static in life and you can change.

From the many people who have attended the Slim by Suggestion sessions, we have come to know that, VERY broadly speaking, there are three key personality types who attend. There is the highly stressed individual whose stress levels just add to the emotional turmoil around weight issues; there are the highly emotional participants, and it is their sensitivity which just adds more turmoil to their other unconscious triggers when they try to deal with their weight; and there are the individuals who just do not know how to behave around food, due to old beliefs and behaviours. It is some of these participants who have said the following at the end of the programme. If they can, you can.

'I have learned so much about why I reach for food when I am upset or bored or lonely. Roz and Georgia really understood why we overeat or get out of control. It's a start, but feeling positive is great.' *Jane, 49*

'Food is no longer a major issue. I'm very relaxed and have dispersed my feelings of guilt. It has revolutionized my way of thinking and dealing with food and diets. I've rarely felt so good losing weight.' *Celia, 42*

'I really enjoyed all the "psychology" behind our relationships with food. I was down one dress size in the first four weeks. When you realize how your patterns of thought restrict and define you, and learn how to change them, weight loss is so much easier.' *Kathryn, 29*

'The programme was superb and easy going – I very much like the no scales and at-ease attitude.' *Juliet, 24*

'A programme which is well thought out, gives invaluable advice and help and makes you feel like a new person.' *Ellie, 36*

'I joined the programme out of desperation. By the end I realized I wasn't desperate at all, it was just how my mind used to think. I have lost 18 pounds.' *Felicity, 31*

About You

'The biggest influence on my eating patterns since my mother!' *Katie, 42*

'It makes you aware of why you're eating. It's a good long-term solution for weight control.' *Alice, 28*

'An excellent programme which delivers what it promises. You must be committed to it – but if you are, the results are excellent. The CD makes it all so much easier.' *Caroline, 35*

'Roz and Georgia taught me how to develop the right mind tools to release the weight that I had been carrying for too many years.' *Tim, 40*

'It was good to realize that there are people out there with the same problems as myself and accept that there IS a solution.' *Laura, 34*

'Slim by Suggestion feels like the weight comes off your mind.' *Dan, 32*

These are some typical remarks that participants make during the eight-week programme:

- Feel they are finally in control of their eating.
- Do not have the same fear about putting on weight.
- Are not frightened of reducing their weight.
- Have the confidence to be assertive around people who like to try and sabotage their need to lose weight.
- Sleep better.
- Deal with stress better.
- Emotionally more balanced.
- Deal with change more confidently.
- Don't think about their weight, food and eating as much.
- Feel and behave more confidently.

7
Making a Strong Start

You have already started the Slim by Suggestion programme by reading the preceding chapters and listening to Track 1 on the CD. If you have been attempting all the 'things to try' and making changes in your thinking and behaviour, you will have done some excellent groundwork. Some of the information from the 'About You' questionnaires in Chapter 6 will have helped you recognize your strengths and weaknesses, and identify old habits and behaviours you will find helpful to leave behind.

> To embark fully on the programme, you will need to take all of the steps outlined in this chapter, and guard against old behaviours and negative thinking.

Ten Easy Steps to Weight Loss without Willpower

STEP 1: LISTEN TO TRACK 1 ON YOUR CD

Ideally, you will have listened to this track once or twice a day for at least six days before starting the steps below. All the instructions are on the CD. To get the most out of it, you should listen while sitting comfortably or lying down in a warm place, where you will be undisturbed. The more you can be consistent with twice-daily use, the better support you will receive from your unconscious mind towards achieving your goals. There are a further three tracks for you to listen to. It is important that you read the chapters and listen to the recommended CD tracks in the order they are presented, and allow the specified time to elapse between each chapter/track. It is important to DO, that is, take the action required for you to make the changes you desire.

STEP 2: RECOGNIZE AND NEGOTIATE WITH YOUR INNER CRITIC

Be aware that The Inner Critic is not your personality. Don't allow The Inner Critic to go unchallenged, even though it may feel like a constant dialogue. It will change with you being consistent and listening to the CD.

STEP 3: UNDERSTAND THE ROLE OF THE PERFECTIONIST IN YOUR LIFE

Discover why The Perfectionist has held you back, and use all the techniques to create a new relationship with this inner voice. Choose to use its very positive aspects.

STEP 4: DISCOVER AND UNDERSTAND YOUR PLEASER

Your Pleaser will have a big impact on your behaviour, and consequently your behaviour around food and drink. Negotiate with it and remember the most important person to please is you.

STEP 5: USE LANGUAGE TO REINFORCE NEW, DESIRABLE PROGRAMMES IN YOUR UNCONSCIOUS

You are eating healthily and you strongly desire to lose excess body fat. Deleting 'diet' and 'weight' words from your internal and spoken vocabulary will be working in the right direction to reprogramme your unconscious mind. You are not doing what you may have done before – this is different.

STEP 6: EMBARK ON A HEALTHY-EATING PROGRAMME

You are likely to know that, in order to lose excess body fat, you will need to eat less and exercise more. Choose a healthy-eating programme that lowers your total calorific intake, and make a commitment to yourself to apply its recommendations to what you are consuming.

If you have a medical condition, you must consult your GP before making any changes to your lifestyle. Your GP will be able to give you information about healthy-eating programmes, and many have nurses at the surgery who can support you. Suggestions for healthy-eating plans can also be found in books, magazines, newspapers and websites. *See Chapter 14* for further references on healthy eating.

> Do not eat too little. If you don't eat enough, your body will think you are starving it and will hang on to its reserves of body fat.

If you are tempted into this type of behaviour, you need to make sure you are using your Emotional Journal (*see Step 9*) to consider your deeply held beliefs. Think, too, about what the results of questionnaires meant for you.

It is also important to note that you will not be able to metabolize excess body fat out of your system if you drink less than two litres of water per day. Coffee, tea, fruit juice and alcohol do not count as water. In fact, you will have to drink more water if you consume these drinks. A rule of thumb is that you will have to drink two cups of water in addition to your two litres for each drink of coffee, tea, fruit juice or alcohol. Remember, too, that coffee and tea contain caffeine and alcohol contains sugar, and these can make your stress levels rise and affect you emotionally. Alcohol can lower your inhibitions – from the programme's point of view, this can mean that your Inner Dialogue will become very powerful, reducing your ability to negotiate with your suppressed parts!

From this point on, we suggest that you do not get on the scales. You already know what size you are. Jumping on and off the scales is unhelpful to you. It is probably compulsive behaviour and it may demotivate you. It will certainly activate your Inner Critic and you are back to the talking scales syndrome.

You will need to guard against the type of thinking that comes from your Inner Dialogue, which is designed to keep you where you are now:

The Inner Critic: You're so hopeless at everything, you'll never be able to keep it up, so you might as well indulge yourself with food/drink now.

Response: Thank you. I'll choose what I want to eat or drink and how much.

The Perfectionist: Well, you weren't supposed to have that. You've blown it now. You just can't get it right so you might as well go back to how you were before.

Response: Thanks. I've been pleased with what I've achieved so far. [Remember, this is what you say, even if on some level you are not.] I don't have to adhere to a plan rigidly, so long as I'm choosing to eat healthily.

The Pleaser: You're going to have to gorge yourself because, if you don't, they will think there's something wrong with you, that you don't like their food/drink and you don't like them.

Response: I know that you are my Pleaser part talking and I am going to continue to eat healthily as it makes me feel better physically and emotionally. I choose my behaviour for this occasion.

There are two things the programme believes are important to take on board before you commit to the healthy-eating programme. The first is that people are generally so busy with their own Inner Critics and other suppressed parts that they are too worried about themselves to notice anyone else. So how can everybody be noticing you and what you are eating/drinking and how you are behaving? We say 'it's none of your business what anyone else is thinking'. Say this to yourself if you feel under pressure.

The other cornerstone belief is

'a lapse is not a collapse'.

If you do eat/drink and generally consume over and above what you had planned, then so what? What is the worst that could happen? Someone finds out? It takes you longer to get to your goal? You stay the same as you are? Truly, the worst thing that could happen is that you allow The Inner Critic and The Perfectionist to have their field day and you completely stop the programme. They will have put you back where you were. Re-read Chapters 1 to 6. So if you have a lapse, then that is what it is – a lapse from which you can learn something about your behaviour and what the experience meant to you emotionally.

So decide which healthy-eating plan you are going to undertake, and begin. Be nice to yourself. This is for you, your confidence, your health, your self-esteem – it is not supposed to be a punishment. You can be proud to have made a decision and started Step 6.

STEP 7: KEEP A SLIM BY SUGGESTION HEALTHY-LIVING DIARY

This Diary is to help you understand what you are consuming each day, where, when and with whom. On page 99 there is a sample Diary page for you to photocopy or create in your own notebook or on your computer. There is a column in the Diary for you to record how hungry you truly felt. As we say, if you are eating for a reason other than physical hunger, then you need to look at the triggers that make you consume when you don't really need or want to.

Sometimes it is very instructive to look at exactly what is happening in terms of patterns of behaviour and the emotions that go with them. For instance, if you find that you have to eat something mid-afternoon – and it happens to be sweets, crisps, buns, doughnuts – you may find there is a pattern. If you do this at work, it could be emotional in the sense that you may be using the unwanted food to push down the stress you are feeling. If you do this at weekends, too, there may be something unbalanced about your blood sugar levels, and you are recommended to look at some of the references for information in Chapter 14.

Everyone can learn something by keeping a Healthy-living Diary. It may be about your emotions in connection with food consumption; a pattern of habitual behaviour which you don't need any more; or about your reaction to certain situations or people. You may discover that you need to become more informed about how to eat healthily!

Slim by Suggestion Healthy-living Diary

Write down exactly what you consume every day – all food and beverages (including alcohol). It is an important part of the programme to do this during the day and then reflect in your journal at night.

How to complete each day:

Date :_____

Time and hunger?	Where and who with?	What doing?	What & amount?	How do you feel?
What time is it when you eat or drink? How hungry are you? **1** – Not hungry at all. **2** – Feeling sort of hungry. **3** – Definitely hungry for some time. **4** – Very hungry. **5** – Extremely hungry.	Where are you? *i.e. home, work, train, car, walking etc.* Who is eating with you or is with you while you are eating?	What are you doing before, during and after food? i.e. taking a break from work for 15 minutes or snacking at desk and continuing to answer telephone.	What are you eating and how much? Be honest – this is only for you!	What are you feeling at the time of eating? *i.e. stressed, relaxed, bad mood, frustrated, calm etc.*

Comments: *This section is for you to record anything that is important to you. It may have nothing to do with food but is relevant to how you are feeling.*

CD Track Yes____ No _____   **Journal** Yes ____ No ____
Exercise *Did you exercise today and, if so, what did you do?* _____

Healthy-living Diary

Date :_____ Name : _____

Time and hunger?	Where and who with?	What doing?	What & amount?	How do you feel?

Comments:

CD Track Yes____ No _____
Journal Yes ____ No ____
Exercise _____

STEP 8: EXERCISE MORE!

The majority of diet plans and diet experts insist that exercise is essential if you want to lose weight. The reason is that you will lose body fat if you TAKE IN LESS FUEL OR EXPEND MORE ENERGY or, ideally, a combination of both.

We suggest that you do not join a gym and do not go out jogging. You will be tempted into that syndrome where you do too much and then feel physically so unfit and stiff that you will totally demotivate yourself. We suggest you do undertake 20 minutes of exercise, three times a week minimum. Please don't force yourself to pound the streets jogging, ride an exercise bike for miles or sweat it out at the gym and make the whole thing a hateful chore. You don't have to do it perfectly; you just have to do it consistently. You CD tracks will help motivate you.

You can consider exercising for the purely selfish reason that you want to feel fit and healthy and enjoy life more. In conjunction with your healthy-eating plan, you'll find you have more energy and will actually want to do more physical activity.

Please start gradually and don't overextend yourself.

Make exercise a natural, pleasurable part of your life.

You could choose an exercise video – many of the beginner programmes are 20–30 minutes long – or incorporate brisk walking and taking the stairs as part of your healthy lifestyle. You could choose sociable activities such as yoga, bowling, dancing, tennis and swimming sessions. There are many options. If you allow your body image to stop you, you are using an excuse, and you should think about this – if so many people are negative thinkers (and they are), then they will be too busy worrying about and having Inner Dialogue with themselves to notice anything about you! Go for it!

STEP 9: KEEP AN EMOTIONAL JOURNAL

Keeping an Emotional Journal is an integral part of the programme as it is a valuable learning tool. You are requested to use your personal Emotional Journal to keep a daily record of your progress. It also provides the benefit of giving you time to focus on yourself. You are encouraged to actually think about *you* and how *you* are feeling and behaving for a regular 10 to 15 minute slot each day. We suggest that you use it to comment and reflect upon all or any of the following:

- What you have learned from any of the chapters – what appealed to you, how the information applies to you, what you will consider doing as a result of the suggestions and steps.
- You might like to write about your experiences with the CD tracks (you are encouraged not to talk to anyone else about this as it is your programming for your mind and responses are highly individual).
- There may be situations during the day that test your eating behaviour. You can use the journal to analyse and reflect on what you felt and how it went.
- You may discover aspects of other people and your relationships which require some thought. Writing it all down can really clarify thinking.
- You may have a particularly stressful day and decide to write all about it (you can choose to reflect in your Journal rather than venting your feelings in any other behaviour i.e. kicking the cat, shouting at the children or eating inappropriately).
- You can use the Emotional Journal in conjunction with your Healthy-living Diary – look for patterns in your eating behaviour, for instance.

Making a Strong Start

- Use the Emotional Journal to encourage yourself – pat yourself on the back.
- 'Control of the emotions and behaviour is usually only achieved by understanding and correcting negative experiences, and using the experiences to go forward' – the most important thing is the way you manage to modify your behaviour.

Some people use their computer, some a bedside diary, some a portable notebook, but everyone says how helpful it is to use it. Remember, it's for only eight weeks. It creates an opportunity for you to spend quality time with yourself.

Emotional Journal

(Record that you have completed today's reflections in your Healthy-living Diary.)

DATE:_____

STEP 10: COMMIT TO THE PROGRAMME

Decide to start the programme strongly, today. There is a contract for you to sign. This will outline the elements of the programme you need to undertake to benefit. Signing your name will signify to your mind that this is what you truly desire and will affirm your commitment to yourself. Congratulate yourself – this is a different approach, a whole-person programme.

Slim By Suggestion Contract

```
Name _____
Start date_____
```

1. The participant hereby agrees that he/she is physically and emotionally well to participate in the Slim By Suggestion weekly programme, and that he/she has no medical conditions or is participating in any medicinal course that may interfere with the progress of the Slim By Suggestion programme.
2. The participant hereby agrees to eat/drink in such a way as to constitute 'healthy eating' at an appropriate calorific level to achieve weight loss, and record their consumption daily as part of a Healthy-living Diary, in conjunction with:
3. Exercising for 20 minutes, three times per week.
4. Listening to CD tracks as recommended and, where possible, consistently once or twice each day.
5. The participant hereby agrees that he/she will participate in all of the 10 steps to benefit fully from the concept and techniques used.

I confirm I have read and understood the terms and conditions of the above contract:

Signature _____ Date _____

How to Progress through the Programme

Start your Healthy-living Diary today. You can also record the exercise you did and that you listened to your CD – it will help to keep you on track. Spend some time on your Emotional Journal. For the next six to seven days, listen to Track 2 on the CD.

After six or seven days have elapsed where you have been consistent, read Chapter 8. Information in all the chapters is important, and you are advised to think hard about what the content means to you and to use your Emotional Journal to reflect on any thoughts you have. Continue with all the steps of the programme and CD Track 2 for another six to seven days.

Read Chapter 9. Continue with the 10 steps and listen to Track 1 or 2 on the CD. After six to seven days, read Chapter 10, and progress with all the steps of the programme whilst listening to Track 3 on the CD.

After a further six to seven days of consistent progress with the steps, read Chapter 11, and again, listen to Track 3 on the CD. Move on to Chapter 12 and Track 4 after six to seven days, followed by Chapter 13 using Track 4.

The following chart will help you plan your progress through the programme. We recommend that you follow the programme as described. If you cut corners or rush, you may well be skipping over important material stored in the unconscious which will sabotage or block you from progress. It's taken a lifetime to acquire all your beliefs and attitudes, so a few weeks reprogramming using all the steps of the programme isn't too long.

Read Chapters 1–6	Listen to Track 1, once or twice a day	
Read Chapter 7	Listen to Track 2 Emotional Journal Healthy-living Diary Healthy eating and exercise	6/7 days
Read Chapter 8	Listen to Track 2 Emotional Journal Healthy-living Diary Healthy eating and exercise	6/7 days
Read Chapter 9	Listen to Track 1 or 2 Emotional Journal Healthy-living Diary Healthy eating and exercise	6/7 days
Read Chapter 10	Listen to Track 3 Emotional Journal Healthy-living Diary Healthy eating and exercise	6/7 days
Read Chapter 11	Listen to Track 3 Emotional Journal Healthy-living Diary Healthy eating and exercise	6/7 days
Read Chapter 12	Listen to Track 4 Emotional Journal Healthy-living Diary Healthy eating and exercise	6/7 days
Read Chapter 13	Listen to Track 4 Emotional Journal Healthy-living Diary Healthy eating and exercise	6/7 days
Maintenance	Re-do the questionnaires contained in Chapter 6 and evaluate your progress. You can reread any of the chapters and listen to any of the CD tracks.	

Make a strong start. This is a programme where the support from the
CD will make the seemingly difficult so much easier.

8
Belief Systems

This chapter concerns your beliefs.

Earlier we talked about the excuses we use, those thoughts or inner vocalizations that are self-limiting and can prevent us from moving forward. Remember, your mind will ALWAYS check to see what it knows about a particular thing. It will also trigger the associated emotions, the physical reactions and behaviour in response to what your mind discovers from its search. Excuses are protective and defensive in nature and work alongside your Inner Dialogue – those strongly defensive parts of your personality with real internal voices to keep us toeing the line. Underpinning both are our deeply held beliefs, most of which are stored in our unconscious mind.

These are often called Belief Systems. Imagine your brain as a computer. It will need an operating system to work it, like Windows. Our beliefs function very like programmes that work our brain and thus our emotions and behaviours.

Beliefs – What are They?

Beliefs can be described as opinions we believe to be true. Many of our beliefs are not based on fact or supported by evidence. 'Fat people are jolly', for example – this is just not true. We can gain beliefs, like our Inner Dialogue, very early on, and pick up lots more as we go through each life stage. Well-known examples are 'mother knows best', 'you must eat your greens to be healthy', 'you'll get a cold if you go out with wet hair', 'children are a blessing', 'everyone gets middle-age spread'.

Your belief system is the window through which you see the world. Beliefs determine what you see and how you react to it. They are deeply held inner guiding principles, created and supported by our unconscious mind, which we constantly reinforce in our everyday experiences.

How Beliefs Operate in our Lives

Your unconscious mind always takes your thoughts, feelings and behaviour in a direction that supports your internal belief system. If you attempt to do something, like lose weight or get fit, and that is in conflict with your inner beliefs, then you will step into a battleground of conflicting ideas.

> If you were told that it was normal to accept second helpings and rude to refuse them, your behaviour will conflict with your desire to eat healthily.

Your thoughts may be 'My host will be upset if I leave any of the meal/don't have second helpings'. Or 'Healthy eating is embarrassing in company' or

'I'd better eat normally (i.e. a lot) because I don't want to draw attention to myself'. So it's OK to keep eating then. Your belief was stronger than your desire, and your mind created any excuse to get you to support the belief.

If one of your beliefs concerns age, for instance, 'I am too old to change', then that is accepted by the unconscious as true. Your unconscious will agree with this concept and manifest it for you. Your attempt to lose weight or get fitter will ultimately not lead to the change you desire – your desire will be in conflict with your belief. Some people may even experience this conflict through physical symptoms which will prevent them from getting fitter. Others may have an overwhelming sense of hopelessness or depression which will 'block' them from their goal. The unconscious mind believes in your beliefs – until you change them.

Identifying and changing your central beliefs is an important task to undertake and is the way in which to achieve your true potential and positive outcomes. Once you can identify your personal self-limiting beliefs, you can reprogramme them so that you are not held back from achieving your goals. Track 1 on the CD will already have helped. Now it is time to listen to Track 2 for a further six to seven days. It will help you achieve this both consciously and unconsciously.

It is likely that you will have plenty of beliefs concerning food – here are the top 10 from the Slim by Suggestion groups:

1. Eating healthy food is boring.
2. It's too time-consuming to eat healthily.
3. You must eat everything on your plate – other people/starving children would be grateful for ...
4. Dieting makes you fatter.
5. It's not fair.
6. Why should I have a weight problem? I hardly eat anything.
7. People in my family tend to be overweight.

8. I don't want to draw attention to myself by eating healthily at social functions.
9. People should love me for who I am, not what I weigh.
10. My boyfriend/girlfriend/partner/wife/husband doesn't mind my size, so why should I have to bother?

Consider other beliefs mentioned here. You can use your Emotional Journal to examine some of your personal beliefs and to record beliefs that 'pop' into your mind over the next week. We cover lots of areas where beliefs are strong so that the whole network of your belief system has a chance to shift and change where necessary. If a belief is stored so that you don't realize it is affecting you, then you may find yourself feeling unaccountably stressed or emotional, and you could be vulnerable at that point to use food or drink to push down the feelings.

PARENTAL INFLUENCE

- A mother should be at home.
- A father is always at work.
- Men talk down to their wives.
- Men don't cry.
- You can't be loved because you didn't do as you were told.
- You are always clumsy.
- You father wouldn't approve of that.
- You are a stupid child.
- Nice girls don't ...
- You are horrible because you are always getting so messy.
- People from our family don't get on in the world.
- Other people have it better than we do.

PEER GROUP INFLUENCE

We get many of our beliefs directly from others. For example, a bad experience at hospital for one child can mean a whole class of children believe hospitals are bad. Sometimes we have copied or aped another's behaviour because we believe a benefit will come our way.

- If I am ill I will get the same attention as my sick sister.
- Hospital was really scary – they use needles.
- They always get what they want, I never do.
- If I give away my toys and sweets, they will like me.
- Everyone at school says I'm thick.
- You are not as good as me.
- Your cousins are much better at everything.
- I went to the dentist and it was terrible and painful.

MUSICAL INFLUENCE

Music can be very good at triggering emotions. Just think of a tune – the theme to one of your favourite children's programmes, a school hymn, the song you and a lover shared. Does certain music affect you more than other styles of music?

- I am a punk – therefore I have none of my parents' values.
- Rock 'n' roll is the influence of the devil.
- You should like classical music.
- An opera is better than a musical.

MEDIA INFLUENCE

Television, films, newspapers, books and magazines influence our attitudes, as do the personalities and celebrities that are featured as our role models. Equal emphasis is given to people and lifestyles – be they lifestyles to aspire to or lifestyles that are a bad influence. Footballers, pop stars, films and film stars, celebrity parties, drug taking, smoking, dress sense and physical appearance are all under the spotlight. The whole world is aware that Oprah Winfrey has struggled with her weight; Mel C from the Spice Girls was really hurt when everyone commented on her weight gain in comparative pictures. If you are a teenager, you may well be influenced by these images and aspire to a certain way of life. If you are an adult, you may be able to look at the situation with an adult viewpoint and not be influenced. Have you considered how the media influenced you when you were susceptible? Are these influences still being carried around unconsciously?

DREAMING

Dreams are very powerful. There is a theory that they are our unconscious thoughts making themselves known. They may also represent the processing of information from the short-term to the long-term memory. In doing this, your mind will check with your beliefs and new information will need to agree with the current framework of the unconscious before being stored. Dreams – and day-dreams – help to reinforce your belief system in the unconscious mind.

THOUGHTS

Thoughts are under your control; they are not free-floating. Thoughts will attract and attach themselves to other thoughts and associate themselves with similar thoughts, information, emotions, experiences and behaviours.

If your belief system says 'I am not successful at anything', then your thoughts will agree with that belief and create it in reality. Your thoughts are a reflection of your beliefs. Your Inner Critic is very good at constantly reinforcing what we believe: 'I'm so useless', 'I will never be able to do this', 'Yes, it's true, I can never be a success ...'.

FEELINGS

Thoughts and feelings are inextricably linked. When someone says, 'You did that really well', you feel proud and pleased. If you hear a joke, you interpret it in your mind by thinking; then you feel amused, happy and laugh. Check to see if you have been told that there are feelings you should or shouldn't have:

- It is not safe to feel angry.
- Don't show your feelings – never lose face.
- Don't be happy – your sister is very upset.
- That's not funny.
- It's not a laughing matter.
- You should be embarrassed.
- Don't go all weepy and over-emotional.
- That temper will get you into trouble.

EDUCATIONAL INFLUENCES

For many people, schooling will have left its mark and belief systems about your abilities. How many people have heard or told themselves any one of the following and unconsciously accepted it as true?

- You never try hard enough.
- You will never be any good.
- I can't keep up with the work.
- I'll never understand this.
- You'll never make a decent football player.
- You won't get in that college/class/set/team.
- You are not good enough.
- You're not as clever as ...
- If only you would make more of an effort.
- You cannot organize yourself.
- Your concentration span is just too short.

OTHER PEOPLE'S EXPERIENCES

We are remarkably susceptible to other people's advice, suggestions and judgements, even as adults. Listen for attempts to influence your beliefs:

- It's the best book you'll ever read.
- The best record ever by ...
- You just have to see this film. Everyone's talking about it.
- Do you like Chinese? Well, there's a really good Chinese opened on the High Street. You must go to eat there.

Other people tell tall tales which may be taken at face value, particularly by children:

- The aeroplane ride was so bumpy, everyone was sick.
- The boat was engulfed by huge waves.
- In foreign countries the food gave me stomach cramp.
- German shepherd dogs are vicious and they bite.

Other people's beliefs can lead to obsessive compulsive or phobic behaviours, such as the families who all sleep with the light on at night, families who hide when there is thunder, families who wash excessively, check locks etc.

YOUR OWN EXPERIENCES

You will have been influenced by parents, significant adults, television, peers and siblings, among others. Inevitably, you will also have had your own experiences that shaped your belief systems. Where they come from is of little significance today, only that you become aware of them. Self-limiting beliefs are the most common block to making change in your life.

- People will laugh at me.
- Water is scary.
- I'm useless at ...
- I always fail.
- People cannot be trusted.
- Families are a burden.
- Change is difficult.
- I'll never have enough money.

- I can't have long-term relationships.
- The world is hostile to me.
- I'm not loveable.
- Success has a price.
- I can't be perfect at everything.
- I am right.
- Nobody really likes me.
- Life is a disappointment.
- I've always been overweight.

Rosemarie's Story

Rosemarie was a successful businesswoman who travelled a lot and entertained clients. This meant she had regular client lunches and dinners. She was aware that this was how she began to pile the weight on. She told the group that she couldn't bear it when she was dining with 'those women who exist on a lettuce leaf'. She said that she **just had to have** three decent courses, and for good measure, gave a very amusing monologue on how everyone must avoid modern British cuisine. Why? Because it was 'too stingy and had tiny portions with a dribble of coloured gravy'.

Listening to her speak was interesting. Notice her use of strong words. She said she '**just had to have**'. This was clearly a very powerful urge, and she told us how she 'absolutely had to have' anything she wanted on the menu. We asked Rosemarie to describe the feeling she would get if she were told she could only have one course. She was immediately clear that the feeling was one of loss or deprivation, quite a sad feeling. Over the next week, listening to her CD and making a daily entry in her Emotional Journal, Rosemarie made a startling discovery. She described it like a light bulb being switched on in her head. She realized her belief was that, somehow, she would never be able to afford to eat like this again, so she really had to enjoy it. Each decent meal could be her last. She worked through this thought and decided that it was a really old belief centred on the fact that she couldn't be successful, and it would all be taken away from her.

Often your beliefs, once uncovered, can seem incredibly obvious. This is how it was for Rosemarie. As soon as she had found it, she could deal with it. It lost its power. Rosemarie told us that she had been so much more able to deal with her 'restaurant situation', as she described it. She really could enjoy the good healthy things on the menu and didn't have that awful feeling of loss that she used food to suppress.

John's Story

John was a self-confessed binger. He binge ate and binge exercised. He was 33 when he came to the group and felt he had always struggled with his weight. When asked about his history, he revealed he had always been on the chubby side. However, because he loved sport, he managed to keep it 'under control'. His usual pattern was to eat healthily and play sport and his body tone/weight would soon respond. He could be comfortable with himself and felt much more confident about himself when he was eating and exercising normally. This would last for two or three months at a time.

Then he would suddenly find himself, as he described it, 'falling off the wagon'. He would find reasons to miss his exercise and begin to eat excessively, followed by bouts of even more punishing exercise and depriving himself of food. He told the group he could totally understand yo-yo dieting, and how painful the experience was for him. We asked John to consider everything he now knew about belief systems, to use his Emotional Journal and his CD, and to consider any beliefs around eating, exercise and his body image.

He explained to the group that, during the week after the talk about beliefs, he felt particularly blank, and his Emotional Journal was only about mundane stuff. During the following week, however, he and his wife took their new baby to see his mother. He said he felt the hairs on his neck stand up when his mother, who was cooing over the baby, asked if the baby was feeding enough. 'A chubby baby is a healthy baby,' she said. 'When John was growing up, I was always having to make him eat his meals, or he would have been such a thin, sickly boy.'

John had that eureka feeling. 'No wonder I keep crashing off my healthy lifestyle if deep inside is a belief that being a normal size is sickly and unhealthy.' He also really understood that it was someone else's belief system he was indoctrinated with, and declared that there was no way he was going to pass that one through to his next generation.

Speaking to John some six months after the end of the programme, he said the belief system work was a seminal moment. He now can eat healthily and take normal amounts of exercise. He said that he still had to be on guard for those stray thoughts/ excuses but he knew what the unconscious was up to and was able to remind himself that it was only an old, unwanted belief, not relevant for his life now.

He had even talked to his mum about it, and she had said to him, 'Well dear, it's just the way we were all brought up, what with rationing and disease and all that.'

SOME THINGS TO TRY

- Start to try to recognize the beliefs that hold you back and write them down in your Emotional Journal. You may become aware of them much more easily through listening to CD Tracks 1 and 2.
- Try to recognize the symptoms of an unconscious mind/ conscious mind conflict. If something is not going right or you feel blocked, or you feel strongly that you should be doing something else, or actually impelled to do the opposite, then it is likely to be an old belief system at work. They can be very powerful and create a lot of anxiety and disturbance. Look for patterns around these blockages.
- When you are next in touch with your family, listen out for common family values. What are the things you all believe in? What are your 'family' sayings? These are all good sources and starting points to recognizing your beliefs.
- For those of you who have children, think about the things you say to them. Do you ever come out with sayings that your parents or guardians said to you? Do you trot out phrases and think, 'My mother used to say that'? Even when you think to yourself, 'I sound just like my Mum (Dad, Grandma, Auntie Jackie)', you can be sure that a belief system is at work and there is something in what you said that is being passed through the generations.
- When you uncover a belief, just acknowledge it as something you picked up along the way which is no longer useful, and let it go.

9
Goal Setting

Goal setting is fundamental to making any changes in your life. The question to ask is: 'if you don't know where you are going, how do you know how to get there?'. This applies to your physical self as well as to your professional and personal life.

Goal setting is relevant to everything you want to do. When we considered the functioning of the brain, we described how easy it is to give your unconscious mind a mental blueprint or programme that it believes to be true. Rather than just swing along and see what happens, it is much better to give the mind a positive version of events you desire to manifest in your future. It is one of the properties of the mind to move you in a direction – any direction – as long as you are moving towards something.

Maxwell Maltz, the godfather of goal setting, describes the human as a 'goal seeking mechanism' who needs to move towards something, rather than stand still.

> A person without goals is a person who has no direction.

Most of us have met people who just seem to be drifting. They seem to be in a limbo where everything lacks momentum and enthusiasm. These people are often very unhappy; they can be depressed, even suicidal. They are often the moaners and groaners. Nothing is right and they are constantly dissatisfied and 'woe is me'. They are the types who say that 'life is so unfair' and are full of self-pity. They can and do use overeating and drinking to push down their unhappiness and dissatisfaction. Maxwell Maltz also said, 'Man is like a bicycle, while moving forward he has poise and momentum'. And we all know what happens when the bike stops.

It is well-documented in books about goal setting and motivation that successful people have two things in common: they know exactly what they want and they dream about how to get it.

These people are natural goal setters and they do so without any conscious effort. Without needing to know it, they are programming their unconscious mind.

How do they do this unconscious programming? They think about their ambitions and their desires when they are day-dreaming. They think about them before they go to sleep at night and they think about them when they wake up in the morning. They can be described as having a 'dog with a bone' mentality. They just don't understand the word 'no' or the words, 'it can't be done'. They do not imagine failing!

What is a Goal?

A goal is something you want to strive for, to achieve – an ambition or a success scenario. You can and need to positively desire as many goals as you want. It is important to have goals in three areas: physical goals, personal goals and professional goals. Here are some examples:

- Physical – health, healthy eating, exercise, fitness, size and tone, taking care of yourself, hair, hands, feet, sex life, information and learning, new practical skills, classes, dancing. PLUS your Slim by Suggestion goals.
- Personal – family, social, friends, personal growth, increased confidence and self-esteem, learning new skills, being creative, practical skills, hobbies, collecting, children, relationships, design, gardening, holidays.
- Professional – finance, money, work, career, training, qualifications, voluntary work, business, charity.

SOME GOALS YOU ALREADY HAVE

This chapter is to demonstrate to you and to your unconscious mind that you do have a goal-setting mechanism – it is automatic and already operating in your mind. You may not recognize it but your unconscious mind is likely to have goals already installed for you NOT to lose weight. Put it this way – due to your past experience of gaining/losing weight, your mind thinks that this is your goal. So your mind will naturally refer to your unsuccessful attempts and try to deliver the same outcome to you; it thinks the unsuccessful attempts are your goal. You need to reprogramme your unconscious mind and provide it with the imagined experience of a successful outcome. That is what you will be doing in your self-hypnosis through the CD Tracks 1 and 2.

You can think your goals through on a conscious level, but they need to be installed as a programme in the unconscious mind. Any conscious goal setting will be overridden by your unconscious goals. This is the reason why so many people 'fall off the wagon'.

Many people don't have enough positive goals, only have negative ones, and those negative goals, like gaining weight, always seem within instant reach. If I asked you the question about exactly 'how' you were going to lose a stone (6 kilos) in the next two months, what image, what experience, would you pull from your mind? Think about it for a while. Have you really considered how you were actually going to achieve it? Sticking to a healthy-eating programme will be part of your goal, but how about all the other aspects of losing excess body fat, like exercise, and all the new behaviour you will need. Just think for a bit ...

Have you been sitting and thinking (goal setting) about dealing with your stress levels when you have to deal with so many difficult people? Have you got a plan for how you are going to deal with that dinner party? What behaviour will you need when you are in the supermarket? Look at all the potential obstacles that may tempt you to break your Slim by Suggestion programme. Start to think about negative situations and now turn them into scenarios in your mind for dealing with them positively. Being able to say no to certain foods and situations will be necessary, because that is your goal. Yes? To lose excess body fat? Agreed? You will be amazed at the difference to your outcomes if you just sit down and work out a plan. We suggest a daily plan and a forward or weekly plan to encourage things in your life that will support your physical goals.

You can use the time while you are relaxing with CD Tracks 1 and 2 to imagine and plan in your mind how you are going to get there. You can also use your Emotional Journal to set out, in writing, the steps you are going to take. Writing down your daily and weekly plan will consolidate the new programming in your unconscious.

Goal Setting

How to Plan Your Positive Future

As you know, the unconscious mind does not know what is past, present or future. It only knows what you imagine. So in planning and imagining your future, your unconscious mind will automatically think you have already experienced that future. Simply put, all you need to do is to repeat, repeat and repeat the thoughts, images and feelings associated with your goals a number of times a day and the mind will get it. Then it is the job of the mind to make it happen for you.

So in this chapter you can focus on your goals. While listening to CD Tracks 1 and 2, you can start to use your imagination and all your senses to create the new programme you desire. In this way your unconscious mind will get the message. In addition, you can day-dream your goals, as the more you imagine any positive outcome, the greater chance there is that it will happen. It really does work.

The Four Most Important Senses for Goal Setting

We mentioned earlier that using the imagination with the senses is the best way to programme your unconscious mind.

Most people have a sense that is naturally dominant. For instance, if I think about the last time I went on a summer holiday, I would have a picture in my mind that represents that holiday. I could see a scene in my mind's eye. That shows that I use the VISUAL sense primarily. Another person will hear the sound of the sea crashing onto the beach, or the rustle of the trees in the breeze. They will be described as primarily AUDITORY. These types can hear sounds from their memory, words that were said. Another sense that can be triggered is a KINAESTHETIC sense. This is where you will remember touch and sensations: the cold of the sea or the warmth of the sun on your skin, for instance.

Everyone is different and has different combinations. Mainly we hear people talk about 'visualization', and that is fine for people who are primarily visual types. Other types experience their imagination and self-hypnosis through their other senses. It really doesn't matter which sense you use primarily in your imagination to programme your unconscious. Use as many of the senses as you can to make it as real as possible to your mind.

AUDITORY — HOW YOU HEAR THINGS

The art of listening on a conscious level is pretty easy. We can often remember words and phrases that are said to us. Sadly, due to the protective nature of the human mind, we seem to remember the bad things people have said over and above any good things we have heard.

Liz's Story

Liz was finding the goal setting section of the programme difficult. As she was a very successful businesswoman, we all were very surprised. I asked her about her life and if she had planned anything, like her career. She said she couldn't goal set and had never done so. She said that her life had just gone along without any formal planning. I was very suspicious and felt that Liz had a block or some type of resistance. So I asked her what were her thoughts when she had tried to diet before and had she had any plan in her mind? Liz was very thoughtful about the question and said she would get back to me.

The following week she said the penny had dropped and she recognized that The Perfectionist wouldn't allow her to set goals just in case she might fail. Her Perfectionist part was too vocal and, coupled with The Inner Critic, it was impossible for her to set goals in her mind. She said she felt an emotional wreck as all she could hear were conflicting words and statements with all the imagined visual pictures that went with them. Very powerful and effective negative programming!

So each day, while listening to her CD, she rehearsed positive Inner Dialogue with all the positive images and visual references, whilst telling her Perfectionist part that goal setting was OK and that she could lose weight. It took some negotiating but it did work.

We asked Liz to keep repeating positive statements in the present tense to herself, particularly if her Inner Dialogue was intrusive.

So start to be more aware of what you are saying internally. Your conversation to yourself may be what your unconscious mind hears as a goal for it to manifest – and so your Inner Dialogue may actually be sabotaging your goals. For any negative thoughts, in words, that you dream to yourself, you will need to start to say the opposite and override the negative programming.

It may seem too simple. However, talking to yourself about what you want and planning it verbally means that you have a pathway down which to travel, to get somewhere you really want to go.

KINAESTHETIC – TOUCH

People who are predominately kinaesthetic are very touchy, feely types. They have a great love of sensations such as the feel of different fabrics, of the wind blowing against their face, of the sun beating down on their skin in the summer. They also have the ability to associate smells with memories and information. The smell of freshly baked bread, for instance, may remind them of their childhood; similarly, they may have specific associations with other smells, such as the aroma of coffee brewing. Kinaesthetic people are often highly emotionally charged and laugh or cry easily. Being so powerful, this sense can be a great tool to use in goal setting in your imagination.

Start to imagine scenes where you can feel the shape and touch of your clothes (at the size you require, of course), or of swimming with a toned body with the smell of the sea allowing you to feel free, or the coldness of an ice-capped mountain where you are safely alone. Your visual sense will probably kick in to reinforce the feelings and your goals will feel vivid. Feeling good about what you are wearing (even if you are not there yet) will programme your mind to take you there; just give it time and persistence. It will be a lot better than thinking negative thoughts with their consequent negative results.

Pete's Story

Pete had a real problem with (in his own words) the 'touchy, feely business'. I explained to him that often it was difficult for men to be relaxed with this as sometimes they equate touch with sex.

He acknowledged this, and because his partner assumed touch meant sex too, his sense of touch was very suppressed. Pete could see that this was a belief system, and that this feeling and touching sense was something he could use in his imagination as a pathway to get in touch with his own physical body and learn to appreciate it. At the end of the programme, he said relearning this sense had improved his sex life as well as making him feel more confident about being a sensual person. He could day-dream for hours using touchy, feely senses, and it worked really well for him as he shed two stone (12 kilos) in three months.

VISUAL — IMAGINING IN PICTURES

Visualizing any experience is a very effective way of setting goals as your unconscious mind has a great capacity to store images. Being a visual person means that your imagination uses pictures, and when you day-dream your imagery is very clear. Visualizing your goals is a wonderful experience and is a brilliant way to plan anything you want to achieve. Your mind will literally take your imagery and create a reality. So you can start to imagine seeing yourself slimmer, getting that promotion, doing something for you. Bring in the other senses too. In fact, dream anything that you want. The more you imagine the same positive outcome, the stronger the unconscious mind will direct you to it.

EMOTIONS — HOW YOU FEEL ABOUT YOU

Using your emotions – along with your auditory sense, your visual sense and your kinaesthetic sense – will programme your mind in the most powerful way. Whenever you want to set goals, 'feeling' the outcome can make all the difference in your unconscious. For example, try this consciously: think happy thoughts, remember happy incidents, think about what will make you happy. You will find your mood will lift; you will stand taller; smile; your eyes will relax; tension will be released from your shoulders and neck; your body will change its strength and posture. Another benefit is that you will feel good. Conversely, if you think about something sad, then you may want to cry; your shoulders will hunch; there will be increased physical tension; and you will feel the emotions associated with the sad situation you have thought up. More proof that what you think is what you get.

When setting goals, imagining an emotion such as happiness, pride or elation means that you will start to marry the emotions, whatever you choose, with being slim, getting that job or whatever you truly want.

Clare's Story

Clare was quite shocked when she realized that when she imagined being slim, she felt fear. This is quite a common feeling, especially if you have never really been slim. If the unconscious mind experiences the emotion of fear, it will automatically protect you against the feeling and not allow you to go there. So her mind was actually holding her back from being slim. Fear is not an option; it is an experience we all have from time to time to warn us about something. Clare had to process that one by using CD Tracks 1 and 2 and starting to imagine feeling safe being slim. It did take time, but once she acknowledged that the fear was holding her back, she could move on.

Benefits of Goals

- Sense of direction and focus.
- Positive thinking.
- A measurement of how you are progressing.
- A feeling of being on track in your life.
- High self-esteem because you are achieving something for you.
- No procrastination.
- If you find your Inner Critic being vocal – just think about your goals instead; the Inner Critic needs a rest!

Setting Your Goals

There are four important questions you need to ask yourself:

1. What do you need to do in order to achieve your goal?
2. What will keep you motivated to achieve it?
3. How will you know that you have achieved your goal?
4. Is the goal realistic and manageable in your lifestyle?

1. WHAT DO YOU NEED TO DO?

You need to write down the tools you need to lose weight. For example, you need an eating programme that is comfortable for you, so that you can achieve your goal in a safe period of time. You also need to plan time for your self-hypnosis, as well as setting out a daily plan of what you can achieve. You must have a plan of what you are going to do and how you are going to deal with awkward situations.

2. WHAT WILL KEEP YOU MOTIVATED?

You need to keep motivated. Without motivation, it is going to be very difficult to stay on track. You will need to make sure you listen to the CD tracks once a day for a minimum of three weeks. It takes approximately 21 days to confirm a new programme in the unconscious. So go for it. Try and avoid people who demotivate you, any saboteurs lurking around.

3. HOW WILL YOU KNOW YOU'VE ACHIEVED YOUR GOAL?

It may seem strange to ask yourself this question. However, it is a tool for ensuring that you have set a clear goal, with all bases covered. If your goal

Slim by Suggestion

is not clear, you may not feel you are getting anywhere. Write down exactly what you want, so your mind knows what it will be like when you get there. You will know that you have arrived.

4. IS THE GOAL REALISTIC AND MANAGEABLE?

Please make sure your goal is realistic. Don't set something you know you cannot really meet. Be honest. We can guarantee that if you set a goal of losing a stone (six kilos) in two weeks, you are setting yourself up for failure, and your Inner Critic as well as your Perfectionist will kick in and your self-esteem will plunge. If you want to be a rocket scientist and you know you have no qualifications at the moment, then you cannot expect it to happen in one year or even two, as you will have to study to get there. Make your goals as realistic and achievable as you can.

SOME THINGS TO TRY

- Start setting your goals now – don't prevaricate! Look at the list of example goals on page 122. Use this to give you ideas.
- The key questions are: what are your goals and aims? What sensations, pictures, sounds and feelings go with their successful outcome? Think through them consciously. Then work on them while you listen to Tracks 1 and 2 on the CD. It's important to write them down in your Emotional Journal.
- Set a time frame for your goals, and remember to set a new goal when you've nearly reached your current goal! It is a lifelong process that keeps us growing and fulfilled.

10
Assertiveness – All About Communication Skills

This chapter can also be described as being about communication and honesty. A key implication of behaving assertively is that your communication is 'straight'. How many times have you edited what you really want to say, so that you create the 'right' impression or so that the other person won't take offence or feel hurt? Being assertive is about being truthful with yourself about what you want and need; and taking responsibility for your choices. It's about not judging yourself, and about taking your own decisions and actions without your Inner Dialogue, or other people, steering you off course.

Assertive Rights

Assertiveness training started as a behavioural therapy method and was further developed by Karl Rogers in the 1970s, who added the concept of a Bill of Human Rights. Rights are defined as 'something to which you are entitled', and a basic right is the 'right to be assertive'. The concept of rights helps you assess if you are being treated fairly or not. There are many lists of rights. Here are some for you to agree with/disagree with/add your own to:

1. The right to ask for what we want (acknowledging that the other person has the right to say no).
2. The right to have an opinion, feelings and emotions, and to express them.
3. The right to be different, to be an individual.
4. The right to make statements which have no logical basis and which you do not have to justify.
5. The right to make your own decisions and to deal with the consequences.
6. The right to choose whether or not to get involved in the problems of others.
7. The right to say no.
8. The right to a fair hearing.
9. The right to ask others for help.
10. The right to change your mind.
11. The right to be successful.
12. The right to be alone and independent, and the right to privacy.
13. The right to have others respect your rights.
14. The right to make mistakes.

15. The right not to know about something, and not to understand.
16. The right to change yourself and behave assertively.

Assertiveness is about being direct and clear in expressing feelings, needs and wants. Assertive behaviour allows people to communicate and relate to each other in an open and frank way.

To behave assertively doesn't necessarily mean that you get what you want, but it does mean you are not left with unfinished business. You will know unfinished business – it's when a situation occurs and you spend days rewinding the scene and wishing you had said something differently or had acted another way.

If you are not able to say NO or speak up for yourself, you can build up inner resentment and anger towards others and yourself. A common reaction to this is to use food/drink to push these feelings down or otherwise distract yourself from the situation. The overall aim can be described as creating win/win situations for yourself – workable compromises where everyone's needs and rights are met – everyone wins.

Consider the results of your questionnaires from Chapter 6 and what they indicate about you. If you are not assertive, the frustrations this will bring may well have a bearing on how you eat and drink.

You can react to situations in three ways: with assertive behaviour, passive behaviour, aggressive behaviour or a mixture of these. Let's look at these behaviour types in more detail.

ASSERTIVE BEHAVIOUR

When you act assertively, you are choosing how you want things to be. By being aware of your personal rights, acting with self-respect and expressing your own wishes and needs, you are not only building your confidence, but also creating a lasting skill to help deal with difficult or stressful situations. You are able to manage situations and people around food/drinking occasions as you wish them to be.

PASSIVE BEHAVIOUR

Behaving passively allows others to get their own way, even when you don't agree. By not expressing your beliefs, thoughts and emotions, you behave in a way that makes you feel resentful, bitter and often lonely. You do not say what you want and this will lead to others making choices for you. You expect others to read your mind. Passive behaviour avoids conflict and leads to low self-esteem. Other people are likely to manipulate you into going along with their wishes.

The way you behave around food is also dictated by other people, both directly and indirectly. If you are unable to stand up for yourself, it is easy to have other people make your decisions for you, like how much you will have on your plate or if you will have dessert or not. 'John will have some more cake, he's a big lad', and before John can muster up words to protest, a large slice appears in front of him. Then John feels it will be easier just to eat it than to make a scene about it. When he speaks up for himself, John feels he is drawing attention to himself and 'making a scene'. John has been railroaded, and inside he is full of resentment that nobody will let him make a decision for himself. People are used to John being unable to give them a straight 'yes' or 'no' so they tend to decide for him. And so a cycle is set up. John's reaction internally is one of self-loathing and resentful anger, and he uses food and drink to push these feelings down.

AGGRESSIVE BEHAVIOUR

Behaving aggressively means ignoring the feelings and opinions of others and violating some or all of their rights. This aggression is used when you blame others, put others down and force others to do things your way. An aggressive style is when you want to make choices for others and dominate them, sometimes treating them as children. Aggressive behaviour creates in the aggressor low self-respect, poor self-esteem and a need to control others. Other people call them control freaks, and aggressive people have to deal with the fallout from their behaviour – it often takes the form of bingeing or comfort eating or drinking.

MIXED BEHAVIOUR

Many people react in ways that are a mixture of passive, assertive and aggressive. Think about how your style may change to reflect different relationships. Specifically, how do you behave in relation to any of the following groups? Do you notice any differences?

- Immediate family
- Other relatives
- Work colleagues
- Strangers
- People in authority
- Small groups

- Large groups
- Children
- Opposite sex

GETTING TO KNOW THESE BEHAVIOUR TYPES

Each behavioural style is characterized by a certain body language, a particular type of verbal communication, and creates certain consequences – how it will make others feel and react.

	PASSIVE	ASSERTIVE	AGGRESSIVE
Appearance	Apprehensive	Relaxed	Tense
Posture	Collapsed, uncomfortable, shuffle, nod in agreement.	Upright, calm and assured.	Domineering, macho stance, get 'too close' to others.
Eye Contact	Minimal, averted.	Direct.	Staring, narrow and cold.
Facial Expression	Fawning, insincere, unsure.	Responsive, face other, incline head.	Taut, intimidating, bullying.
Hands	Limp, don't know what to do with them.	Relaxed.	Agitated, fists or fingers pointing, fiddling.
Voice	Hesitant, weak and soft.	Confident, warm and expressive.	Strident, loud and demanding, cold.
Feeling	Anxious, ignored, helpless, manipulated.	Confident, self-respect, valued, purposeful.	Superior, controlling, self-righteous.

Assertiveness

	PASSIVE	ASSERTIVE	AGGRESSIVE
Verbal expression	Apologetic words or vague: 'I mean', 'You know', 'Well'. Often silent.	Say what you honestly think. Clear, objective words and statements.	Say what you want, but at others' expense. Use 'you' words and words that threaten, blame or label.

AGGRESSIVE BEHAVIOUR MAKES OTHER PEOPLE FEEL:	
FEELING:	ACTIVITY for passive/assertive
Angry and threatened	Resent aggressor's unfair tactics
Frustrated	Waste of energy defending themselves from abuse.
Withdrawn	Avoid aggressive people due to the fact they have to be on their guard.
Anxious and defensive	Unable to relax with aggressor around; when is next attack?
Resentful	Resent the power an aggressor has over them.
Hurt	Can't help being hurt by comments and put downs, even though not fair.
Humiliated	Dislike being made to look stupid/ridiculed/corrected in public.
Exhausted	Being constantly on guard is tiring.

Slim by Suggestion

PASSIVE BEHAVIOUR MAKES OTHER PEOPLE FEEL:	
FEELING	ACTIVITY for other people
Aggressive	Shun or avoid passive people, can walk over them again and again.
Irritable	Wish that passive would stand up for themselves and make some decisions.
Distance and avoidance	Avoid the negative attitude of a passive person, don't bother with them, let them 'get on with it'.
Superior	Respect is too difficult when person does not stand up for their beliefs.
Exhausted	Valuable energy wasted in dealing with defeatist/negative attitudes.

ASSERTIVE BEHAVIOUR CAN MAKE OTHERS FEEL:	
FEELING:	ACTIVITY for passive/aggressive
Positive	Sense that an assertive person is supportive with positive attitude.
Secure	Assertive is trustworthy, because others know where they stand.
Co-operative	Can elicit help from others because there is no game playing or point scoring.
Respectful	Reciprocate the respect an assertive person shows for others' needs/rights.
Energetic	Can behave constructively without wasting energy on defence/avoidance and spotting game plays.

Assertiveness

Styles of communication and behaviour can be characterized:

PASSIVE	ASSERTIVE	AGGRESSIVE
Hope you will get what you want.	Ask for what you want clearly and specifically.	Try to get what you want at any cost.
Squash your feelings.	Communicate directly and openly.	Use any method to get what you want.
Rely on others to guess what you want.	Communicate appropriately.	Threaten, bully and use sarcasm or fight.
Agree with opinions that are not your own.	Ask confidently without anxiety or apprehension.	Manipulate and cajole, use crocodile tears.
Unable to ask for what you want.	Don't knowingly violate other people's rights.	Blame others.
Never express your own feelings and thoughts.	Look for the win/win outcome of situations.	Get tense and shout to deal with situations.
Never upset anyone.	Communicate and behave confidently.	Use disrespect and dishonesty to violate others' rights.
Don't get noticed.	Negotiates.	Unable to negotiate.

As with most things in life, you will need to practise assertiveness skills so that you can behave assertively in all situations. Begin to consider the following (use your Emotional Journal if you like):

- Where has any lack of assertiveness caused you difficulty and stress?

- Where has aggression or passivity caused you difficulty and stress?
- In which situations or areas would you like to use assertive skills?

Remember, learning a new behaviour takes practice. Start with the easier situations, rehearse them mentally, talk them through with a friend, feel good about what you are trying to achieve and recognize it may not go as you wish at first – each practice is a learning opportunity.

Linda's Story

Linda was a dynamic personality but her lack of clear communication led to much frustration. She became very overweight because people would not do what she wanted. Her requests seemed reasonable to her, and when the SBS group questioned her communication style as being aggressive, she was adamant that she wasn't: 'I'm not aggressive'.

Some weeks later, whilst listening to her CD, she realized that people in her workplace were avoiding contact with her because she was aggressive. Around seven years previously, Linda had been the victim of a mugging just outside her office. This was a very traumatic and upsetting incident. Linda came to realize, through her Emotional Journal and by monitoring her thinking, that she was particularly anxious when she felt her personal control was being violated.

Linda began to take control of her own behavioural responses and her thinking so that each approach at work was a negotiation rather than a threat to her personal domain. Linda will tell you it wasn't easy and that it was a case of taking one day at a time. In this way, she began to learn what was within her control and what was outside her control.

A great benefit of this was that she was focusing so much on her behaviour and her emotional responses that the amount of time she spent thinking about food and eating lessened considerably. She commented, 'Now I am not avoiding my emotions about the mugging, I don't need to think about food all the time.' She realized that she had focused her whole world on food and eating because dealing with the mugging and its effects was too painful.

Karen's Story

When Karen starting attending the programme, she was extremely aggressive and hostile. She constantly interrupted the lectures, and each week would have a tale to relate about a drama going on in her personal life. As the weeks unfolded, we learned something more about the relationship with her live-in boyfriend. The boyfriend would react to any request she made by purposely doing the opposite. For example, lying in bed all day when it was his turn to do a chore. She would be aggressive towards him all weekend. She said 'He makes me so angry because he never does anything I want him to do. I say black, he says white.'

You may think Karen should have got rid of him. However, once she learnt to be more assertive in her requests, rather than aggressive and domineering, he was more than happy to do things. She recognized the power of being assertive as opposed to aggressive, and that a win/win situation was possible. Once their communication was clear and without anger and manipulation, they discussed how the relationship could be saved and were glad that the mutual attraction they had remembered from the beginning was still there.

Karen's assertiveness skills gave her another benefit: she could now communicate more assertively at work. She realized that other

people have a choice about how they want to react and that
you cannot demand a response that is just the one that you want,
just because you want it. Once she had come to terms with that,
she acknowledged how much her eating had been to push
down feelings.

Assertiveness Skills

There are many good books available on assertiveness, which you may find
useful. The following is a list of the main assertiveness skills. You can use
them in conjunction with the behavioural skills detailed in the tables on
pages 137–140, such as eye contact, posture, firm handshake, clear voice
and confident approach. Your CD will help you too.

BE SPECIFIC

Decide what you want or need and say so directly and specifically. Avoid
unnecessary waffle and speak briefly and simply. This skill will help you to
be clear about what you want to say and your positive outcome.

USE REPETITION

You may have heard of a technique called 'Broken Record'. This skill helps
you to stay with the clear statement or request you have rehearsed. Repeat
yourself calmly and you will be able to hold your clear and specific position
without being manipulated or distracted by someone else who has a
different agenda. They may try logic or confrontational argument to get

you to move from your position away from your wishes. If you are saying NO, you may have to repeat it a few times before the message is heard. Tell them your reasons if you feel there is a need to do so. You don't owe anyone an explanation. Stay calm and breathe deeply to reduce any anxiety.

HOW TO MAKE A RESPONSE

Good communication involves listening to others and acknowledging what they have said, even if you don't agree or it is manipulative. You need to let the other person know that you have heard their comment or opinion – without getting caught up with what they are saying. When a request is made, repeat and précis what is being asked of you, clearly and to the point – cut through any padding around the request.

NEGOTIATING THE 'I WIN/YOU WIN TOO' POSITION

When there is a conflict between the needs and wants of the involved parties, you will need to take both viewpoints into consideration, honestly. Find the true compromise or the solution to the problem by clear communication, asking questions and direct responses. If you cannot find an immediate compromise, agree to both think about it and agree on a time to discuss it again. You have the right to refuse any request, to buy thinking time, to walk away from aggression. Don't respond with an habitual apology.

EXPLAINING YOUR FEELINGS

This allows you to express your feelings with a simple statement, such as 'I feel nervous', 'I feel guilty' or 'I feel under pressure'. Once you have outlined your feelings about a situation, you will be able to relax more, dispel anxiety and deal with it. Just admitting it clears the air and allows you to move on. Other examples are: 'I have made my decision and there is nothing you can say that will make me change my mind.' 'I can see you are trying to make me feel guilty for saying NO, but the answer is no and I am not going to feel guilty about it.'

LISTENING

Keep quiet when you have said what you want to say, particularly if it is NO. It is easy to ramble on explaining yourself and making excuses, and then you may be passive! Remember, some people are very clever at getting what they want; listen carefully to what they are saying. You may find that they use a particular tone of voice and way of speaking when they want something or a favour that they know might be refused.

DEALING WITH CRITICISM

Some is fair; much is not. Everyone has the right to express his or her opinion but you do not have to agree with it. Consider the behavioural style of the person being critical. Listen carefully. If you do not understand the criticism, ask them to explain, clearly and specifically. Take your time. Think about what they are saying to see if it is correct. If it is, acknowledge it, and agree with it where appropriate. This will allow you to move forward rather than retreating, hurt and wounded. Ask if they have any suggestions about ways of doing things differently.

If the criticism is unjustified and there are mixed motives, let the person know how you feel about it in a relaxed, calm and considered way. Here are some examples:

- 'I will accept the criticism that is appropriate, such as XXXXX; the rest I will let pass.'
- 'I feel rather hurt, and I will consider what you have said.'
- 'I would like to think about what you have said, and discuss it with you when I can suggest some solutions.'
- 'I want to think about your comments and I will get back to you. When is a convenient time?'

You can ask for further clarification so you can assess if the criticism is hostile, manipulative or constructive. If it is hostile, you can allow the other person to express their honest negative feelings directly, which will improve communication between you, and allow you to choose if and how you interact in the future.

Use tools, such as the Emotional Journal and self-hypnosis, to let go of unjustified criticism, and any emotions and behaviours it triggers. You do not need to get involved with supporting passivity or arguments and conflicts if you do not want to.

Becoming More Assertive

As you become more assertive, you may also find that the dynamics of your relationships change. It may not suit others around you when you change, and when you have the skills and behaviours to get your needs met. On the other side of the coin, others may be delighted that you are not trampling on them and their wishes in quite the same way. People will notice that you have more confidence and are easier to deal with. You might find your social circle increases.

You might like to start to study the behaviour of others by listening to what and how they communicate; it will be very informative!

SOME ASSERTIVE REHEARSALS FOR YOU TO TRY

It can be very helpful to practise being aggressive, assertive or passive. Look at the table on pages 137–8 to see what posture, body language and tone of voice are used in each type of behaviour. Then take an imaginary scene and act out how you will respond in each mode. This is a good way to recognize what each behaviour actually feels like, and you will know when you have slipped away from being assertive into one of the other modes in real life.

Below, there are some suggested subjects for role-playing. You can practise these situations with a friend or on your own. You can add any scenarios you know you haven't handled particularly well in the past, or think of some that are likely to happen in the future. Consider what you will say if any of the following are said to you, and practise the reply/response out loud, bearing in mind your behaviour (eye contact, posture, tone of voice etc.). You can practise being assertive, or pretend you are aggressive or passive:

- I made this dessert especially for you. You must have some.
- Our family always eats well so please don't let the side down.
- I bought you a treat. You like cheesecake normally, don't you?

- I heard you were starving yourself to get so slim. It won't last and you'll put back even more weight ...
- You might as well let yourself go at the buffet party on Saturday, to keep me company.
- You mentioned that you don't eat after 8 p.m. Will you be in a difficult position if I invite you to an important dinner function?
- I made us some sandwiches. Tuck in, there's chocolate cake for afters.
- You look so thin and pale. I liked you when you were happy and jolly.
- Who does she think she is with all that exercising? Miss Perfect?

Rehearsing situations can also be helpful. Say you have a family function coming up and you are expecting comments on what you are or are not eating, you can prepare your responses in advance. Remember to see yourself in your imagination remaining calm and in control in the face of provocation! Maybe it's a job interview, or a special date. Someone may be tempting you with chocolate or alcohol. You can rehearse in your imagination to set your unconscious mind up to see the successful outcome as your goal. In this way you will be able to remain in charge of your behaviour and thinking.

As you consider the information in this chapter and your reaction to it, you can use your Emotional Journal to reflect on your thoughts or on any situation. Take time to think of those successes you have had; how well you did; how your practice attempt went better than expected. Pat yourself on the back – you deserve it.

Listen to CD Track 3 for six to seven days and move on to the next chapter.

11
Anger and You

The word 'anger' carries with it a raft of meanings and associations, mostly unpleasant. The images we receive of anger are of abuse, violence, hurt and fear, and of people who are out of control when they express anger. The emotion of anger is not socially acceptable, and people generally shy away from, or avoid at all costs, any emotion that is considered uncivilized.

This human urge to civilize and be civilized has led to the situation where the emotion of anger is suppressed. For most of us, this emotion was not allowed an outlet when we were children as we were brought up to 'turn the other cheek' and 'forgive and forget'. The expression of anger in tantrums or rage is something that most children are not permitted. Consider your thoughts and reactions the last time you saw a child having a temper tantrum. It can be very uncomfortable just to be near a demonstration of anger, even in a child.

Dealing with Anger

Even with assertiveness skills, anger is hugely difficult to deal with. One reason for this is that we may not even understand what the emotion of anger actually feels like. We normally find that some emotions are easier to deal with than others, and the easiest emotions to express are those that were most accepted and expressed in your household as a child. Every family or group has its own range of emotions within which it operates; some are acceptable and expressed, and others are discouraged or even not permitted. As children, we often substitute an acceptable emotion and behaviour for the real feeling, and do it so often that it becomes automatic. It is then an unconscious reaction and a conditioned reflex. Track 3 on the CD is designed to allow you to deal safely and supportively with these old behaviours and the emotions of anger. This chapter may trigger reactions which you can reflect upon in your Emotional Journal.

HOW WE SUPPRESS ANGER

So, for the emotion of anger we may show external 'niceness': Instead of expressing or feeling anger, we might show an outward sadness or we may demonstrate hostility. We may become fawning or withdrawn, or boisterous or bullying. An angry feeling may make us grit our teeth and think vengeful thoughts.

The problem with substitute emotions is that we are left still carrying the anger around with us – and it gets stored away along with all the other unexpressed anger. This is why it seems so dangerous to get anywhere near the angry state; you won't just be expressing today's anger, because all the unexpressed, stored anger will explode too. This is the reason why suppressing and expressing anger is extremely stressful.

One of the ways that we tend to deal with anger is to, literally, 'swallow' it, pushing down the emotion with food or drink.

You may have noticed through your Emotional Journal and Healthy-living Diary that some situations and people in a way that triggers a binge. Anger can very easily throw us off course and back into old ways. Track 3 on the CD is also designed to allow you to release old, stored angers. Try the following questionnaire to reflect on your experience over the last six months.

HAVE YOU EXPERIENCED ANY OF THESE IN THE LAST SIX MONTHS? Tick yes or no.	YES	NO
Being unable to feel angry, even when you think you have just cause.		
'Going over the top' with rage at the most inappropriate times or places.		
Taking out your frustration on someone or something else.		
Crying, when you might prefer to shout and bawl.		
Being rendered motionless with fury or becoming speechless.		
Getting stuck in a depression when you are grieving for a loss. (This can be for something like a job, not necessarily for a person.)		
Being cowardly and afraid when someone else expresses anger.		
Being unable to control your anger.		
Having fantasies of violent or spiteful revenge.		
Considering going to the doctor with headaches or stress.		

	YES	NO
Using an angry outburst to draw attention to yourself.		
Being aware that others are scared of your angry or frustrated behaviour.		
Using anger when you think you are going lose an argument or dispute, rather than losing face or having to back down.		
Using anger to make others feel guilty.		
Being aware you are stuck in a bereavement process.		
Feeling nauseous and experiencing palpitations with anger.		
Considering that a compulsion/addiction/obsession may be the result of the stress of frustration and anger.		
Experiencing difficulty in resolving conflicts without hurting yourself or others.		
Using anger to manipulate others – they avoid confrontation and so you win the argument.		

When you are at the end of the chapter, check your results. As the state of expressed or suppressed anger is so stressful, you won't be surprised to find out that there are physical and psychological repercussions.

Anger and Physical Health

Anger is bad for your health. It can shorten your life.

Significant research has been undertaken during the last few decades and the effects of sustained anger can include:

- Digestive problems like gastritis, ulcers, irritable bowel syndrome.
- Circulation problems like hypertension, blocked arteries and raised cholesterol, all of which are factors in heart disease.
- Bowel conditions such as colitis.
- Muscular problems, prolonged tension and inflammatory disorders.
- An inability to deal with infection and increased intolerance to pain, which can hinder recovery from serious illness.
- Headaches, sinus problems, skin disorders.

ANGER AND EMOTIONAL HEALTH

Anger is bad for your emotional and psychological health. It can seriously depress you.

Mental health professionals say that anger is linked with depression, guilt, obsessive behaviours and compulsions, phobias and manic depression. Observation on the Slim by Suggestion programme suggests that there are many more emotional dangers from dealing in the currency of anger as well as the inevitable effect on your ability to control what you eat and drink! For instance, low self-esteem, ritualistic behaviour, substance abuse and addictions and paranoia. And, naturally, there will be an ongoing commentary from The Inner Critic – you and your Inner Critic against the hostile and uncompromising world.

Anger screws up your relationships.

In Gael Lindenfield's book, *Managing Anger*, she quotes research about the 14 physiological changes that take place in the states of anger and sexual arousal. They differ by just four.

> If we are keeping a rein on our anger, we are controlling the physiological processes that lead to sexual arousal. This can lead to frigidity or impotence.

It can also mean that spontaneous sexual arousal becomes impossible and that artificial stimulants like drugs, alcohol or fetishes are needed to become turned on. Sometimes angry people can be promiscuous, as a way of expressing anger without realizing it.

When we push down feelings of anger, we tend to push down all feelings. We get cut off from ourselves, and other people, fearing commitment, and are unlikely to have intimate or satisfactory relationships.

ANGER IS NOT BENEFICIAL

To sum up, anger is extremely damaging for you in lots of ways, and it is likely to be the trigger that sends you to the fridge and on a binge. Then you have to deal with the self-loathing and guilt that may go with it! You will remember that a lapse is not a collapse, but when anger is involved, it is all too easy for everything to spiral out of control. That's why Slim by

Slim by Suggestion

Suggestion calls anger 'the tough one'. You will need to start to monitor your feelings and use your Emotional Journal to support you as you use Track 3 on the CD. You may even find that reading about anger is starting to trigger some feelings you would rather not have.

'TOLERATING' ANGER

As you go through the week, be aware that most people find that their ability to tolerate frustration, or the situations that trigger their anger, will fluctuate. Normally, this tolerance will be near the surface, and you will be 'on edge' when you are:

- overtired
- physically exhausted
- hungry
- experiencing hormonal changes, such as PMS, menopause, pregnancy
- recovering from an operation
- recovering from a traumatic incident
- physically craving an addictive substance, such as nicotine, caffeine, alcohol
- under the weather from flu, a virus, an upset stomach
- suffering from pain, like back pain
- in a state of sexual frustration
- on a high from substance abuse (including legal ones)
- on a high, or hyperactive, as a result of stress reactions

So be particularly kind to yourself as you work through the chapter.

Sarah's Story

Sarah had been a slightly chubby kid and now, at 30, was at least three stone overweight and well known as being hot-tempered. She talked about having regular outbursts of anger at family, friends and work colleagues. These, of course, made her feel guilty and afraid. Sarah had clearly identified that after one of her 'vile outbursts' she completely stuffed her face. She said, 'I don't know why I am deliberately aggressive and try to hurt the people I love the most.'

She freely admitted she was drinking too much, too often, to numb the pain and shameful feelings, and was bingeing on whatever 'she damn well wanted'. She was doing this in private, and it was only when she started to explore her behaviour that she recognized that what her friends and family had said was, in fact, true. She was avoiding socializing, just as she had avoided the truth about it.

She made the group laugh when she said that you can have a better binge in private; everyone knew this was true. Sarah was a big personality with a big sense of humour; somehow she had thought herself into a big body to go with it.

What transpired was that Sarah was very angry with herself all the time, as well as angry about being overweight and out of control with her eating. Being around slim people was causing her to feel even more worthless, and her reaction to that thought and feeling was to be angry and lash out. With Sarah's naturally ebullient personality, we were not surprised to find that Sarah's father was a clergyman and she had been brought up in a very prim and proper environment. Of course, anger or anything expressive was certainly not tolerated, so Sarah suppressed it all and developed a habit from childhood of eating her frustrations.

Being a naturally boisterous and funny kid didn't really go down too well in the rectory, so she developed overeating to deal with the stress of the suppressed feelings. The trouble was that these unexpressed feelings of anger kept spilling over, and so the vicious circle perpetuated itself.

Sarah was very reflective for a couple of weeks after the anger session, and this reflection allowed her to acknowledge her self-sabotaging part and that her weight was a very defensive shield for her to hide behind. She felt that everybody in the world was critical of her – of her personality and characteristics as well as her size. As she began to really think things through, she told us she knew her Inner Critic was a real bitch and hard for her to cope with, but understanding her suppressed anger made her realize that it got its energy from the part of her that was highly critical, not just of herself but of everyone. She said, 'It's not other people being critical of me. I'm thinking this stuff myself and The Inner Critic is egging me on ... I don't go out because I put words into other people's mouths that they don't actually say ... and those words make me so unhappy that I stuff myself.'

It took a while but Sarah, with the help of her Emotional Journal and Track 3 on her CD, began to think 'assertive first, and aggressive last'. This was her personal saying that allowed her to interrupt her behaviour. She knows that she will always have a tendency to bottle up her (angry) feelings, and if she does she will be the one to suffer the backlash. As she said, 'Now I have the information, I have the ability to choose.'

Molly's Story

Molly had experienced depression several times. Through the Slim by Suggestion programme, she came to understand that she was and had been very angry with her parents. In her view, they were very controlling people, to the extent that as her father was a successful lawyer, she was expected to become a lawyer too. So she was a lawyer, and she loathed it! In her childhood household, there was no unconditional love; it was conditional upon achievements and being good. She had always pushed her feelings down with sweet treats, and as an adult with lots of binge eating and drinking.

When she began the programme, her legal training meant that she liked the discipline of the Healthy-living Diary, and it didn't take her long to realize that her eating went particularly out of control before, and especially after, any contact with her parents. This included phone calls, visits, social occasions and even supposedly fun things like going to a gallery or the theatre together. Her father had been a very successful partner of a law firm and he was always asking about her promotion prospects, about when she was going to get a pay rise or a high-profile case. It was even worse now he had retired.

Through listening to Track 3 on the CD, Molly had a growing conscious recognition that she couldn't change her parents or what had happened in her upbringing, and that she needed to deal with her own anger and let the past stay that way. Although it was hard for her, she recognized that she lived in the past to some extent. She would mull things over, and was full of old regrets and remorse about things she could not change. She was also conscious that, in many ways, she had been living her life for other people and meeting their needs over her own.

By acknowledging her own behaviour and emotions, particularly the anger and her habitual thinking about blame and regret, she was able to let it go from her unconscious mind using the CD. With her conscious mind and lawyer logic, she was able to see that her reactions of eating and drinking too much when she had contact with her parents were a matter of her own personal choice. She therefore finally felt in control.

About six months after the programme, Molly rang to say that she was very nearly at her natural dress size, 12, without any real effort. She hadn't binged in ages and that her father had actually asked her for some advice. She was so stunned she had to call and share it. Things can really turn around when you have your thoughts and emotions under control!

SOME THINGS TO TRY

Use your Healthy-living Diary to monitor the situations and people that trigger you into an 'angry state'. Record and acknowledge what happens to your thinking and behaviour. You can use your Emotional Journal to work through your issues. Consider the following suggestions as well:

- Monitor your anger – be aware of the thoughts that set off the old patterns.
- You can safely perform anger; you do not need to feel it/let it take over.
- Delay an angry response; take deep breaths. Putting off an immediate out-of-control reaction will put you back in control.
- Think about degrees of anger. It is not appropriate to be 100-per-cent angry – the appropriate response may be cross, frustrated, disappointed, irritated or just pissed off. See the Angry Word Listing on page 161 of this chapter for other adjectives for feelings that may be far more suitable for the

situations you find yourself in. Give the feeling its correct name. It may feel daft but stop, breathe deeply and think, 'I'm actually just about to blow a fuse here, but could the feeling be labelled with another word?' It will feel much safer if you act crossly, disappointedly, let down or annoyed than if you blow into total anger mode.

- Think about disliking the situation, disliking the event.
- Accept that not everybody you meet or associate with will agree with you or even like you.
- Accept that not everybody will behave as you would wish.
- Accept that not everybody has assertiveness skills and not everybody will respect other people's rights.
- Change your expectations of others. If they are unrealistic, you may get disappointed, and your response to disappointment may be inappropriate anger.
- Be aware that being angry is not good for you physically or psychologically. It raises your stress levels.
- When you are not angry, talk with those people you allow to trigger your anger.
- Anger can be expressed at the appropriate level at the right time and to the right person. Gaining control of yourself and your anger levels is an assertiveness skill. Consider, however, whether the object of your anger is worth all the trouble? This may be the right time to move on and to delete the person from your Christmas card list.
- Always remember that you can choose to swallow your anger with food or alcohol! Acknowledge this emotion to yourself as soon as possible.
- Take on simple ways of expressing disappointment, dislike, frustration, unfairness, and irritation – whichever word you

now choose: You can talk to an empty chair about the situation. This is a much better strategy than trying to talk to someone face to face when your anger is out of control. In this way you can say out loud what you really feel. Say what you really think. You can be out of anyone's earshot and alone and be as loud as you like. It will be a cathartic and assertive experience.

- Use your Emotional Journal. You can look at old photos, letters or other mementos that you know have triggered you in the past. Work through them with your new thinking skills (mind tools).
- Thump, pummel or beat a cushion or pillow. Express yourself in words and cry as much as you want to.
- Use Track 3 on your CD and your resolve to deal with those things you know trigger you. You can and will leave them behind, metaphorically, and walk towards a new beginning.

ANGRY WORD LISTING

We commonly use the word anger to describe other emotions – are you really feeling something else?

- fury
- frustration
- pissed off
- resentful
- disappointed

- confused
- fearful
- attacked
- manipulated
- irritated

- annoyed
- taken for granted
- let down
- oppressed
- fed up

If you answered 'yes' to any of the questions on page 151, you may like to consider the fact that not everyone who has had a lousy day, has severe back pain, has the period from hell or has drunk five pints of strong lager will get angry in response to frustration. Also, the state of our health is only part of an explanation for the expression of anger.

If you answered 'yes' to any of the questions, you may like to consider the fact that real anger does not serve many useful purposes, except as a protective surge of energy in a physical emergency. It can immobilize you, physically and emotionally. Performed anger, such as letting a child know it is not behaving appropriately, can be useful but real hot anger is not positive – it can also give others the power to immobilize your emotions whenever they choose. They will know exactly how to wind you up.

If you answered 'yes' to any of the questions, you may like to consider the fact that anger frequently occurs when things do not go the way you want, or people do not respond or react in the way you expect them to. By expressing your anger towards other people, you are denying them the right to see the world in the way they choose. You do not have to like it when things do not go your way, but getting angry will not change things.

As with all emotions, angry feelings and behaviour come from your thoughts – and you may just be triggering old behavioural responses too. If you think different thoughts, you do not need to get immobilized with anger. There is no difference between anger that is suppressed or expressed if you are thinking those same thoughts and replaying old emotional and behavioural patterns.

'The secret of getting rid of the stress of anger is to recognise and accept that people and things will never be exactly how you want them to be. You have no right to demand or expect that others should act in the way that you want them to.' – David Brookes, *Beat Stress from Within*.

12
Finding Your Inner Child

The Inner Child is a very powerful part of you. It is described as the 'vulnerable part' of the Inner Dialogue theory, and it is such a special and important part of Inner Dialogue that it deserves its own chapter. Your Inner Child is within you, and to gain a connection with it can be a very deep exploration of how you really feel and how you have interpreted your childhood. This chapter, and listening to Track 4 on your CD, will provide a safe environment to explore your childlike and primitive Inner Child behaviours and feelings. These are the feelings that are often completely suppressed out of conscious awareness and are mostly unacceptable in the adult world.

There is a huge benefit from making a connection with your Inner Child.

Some of the strong, inexplicable inner urges you experience are likely to be your child trying to be heard.

If your child feels vulnerable or hurt in a situation, even when the adult seems OK, the child will want to push down its feelings through behaviour like tantrums and violent outbursts or through socially acceptable ways like eating and drinking. These instances can be when you feel 'out of control'.

How many of us can say we had a perfect childhood? Some of us had better ones than others. This chapter explains the concepts of the personality traits of The Inner Child and how much they affect us, without much conscious recognition. It will demonstrate to you that you really did the best you possibly could with the limited information you had as a child, and that now you can reconnect with this wonderful part to become a much more fulfilled person.

Inner Child Personalities

All Inner Child traits are raw, emotional and unconditional. It is such a shame that as adults we are not 'allowed' to express these feelings, because belief systems are that adults do not cry, they are not allowed to rant and rave, they are not allowed to laugh and be silly. Adults are 'mature' people and childlike behaviours are judged to be unacceptable. When we are among other adults, we fear allowing our more childlike traits to come out.

The reason why childlike characteristics are suppressed is often the result of family expectations, where so-called 'mature' behaviour is demanded from children before they are ready. Did you experience the belief that 'children should be seen and not heard'? In many families, this literal attitude meant that children were excluded from conversations so couldn't ask questions and explore. They certainly couldn't form relationships with their parents and older people in general.

Perhaps you heard statements such as:

- 'Big boys don't cry.'
- 'Girls are too emotional.'
- 'Grow Up!'
- 'Stop being such a baby.'
- 'You're supposed to set an example.'
- 'You are too old for that now.'

There is a lot of pressure on children to grow up quickly, and sometimes this is at the expense of developing parts of our personality and gaining experience.

Our belief systems are clearly linked to our Inner Child. As we are developing during childhood, we attempt to learn how behave, how to make sense of the world and how to get on in the world. In a way, this is the essence of The Inner Child: it needs to learn quickly how to understand the world and especially how not to rock the boat too much in order to be loved unconditionally.

ADULT/CHILD CHARACTERISTICS

To discover The Inner Child, we can look at the characteristics of an adult, then a child. In the Slim by Suggestion groups, these are the sort of traits that usually come up:

Children	Adults
Spontaneous	Responsible
Fun	Logical
Cheeky	Set in their ways
Demanding	Repressed
Illogical	Rigid and inflexible
Loving	Give conditional love
Open to learning	Educated
Dependent	Independent
Financially dependent	Financially independent
Suggestible	Full of preconceived ideas
Uncomplicated	Complex
Gullible	Paranoid
Live for the moment	Suspicious
Open	Closed
Manipulative	Manipulative
Interested in many things	Pay for fun and leisure
Creative	Unimaginative
Free	Feel trapped
Silly	Stiff upper lip

When you look at the two sets of characteristics, they are virtually opposite. In fact, they could be described as two different people, or are they?

Everybody has an Inner Child, just as everyone was once a child.

For those shaking their heads at the moment, it can mean only one thing – your Inner Child is very suppressed and too frightened to come out. Take another look at the list and ask yourself when was the last time you displayed some genuinely and spontaneously childlike traits? We all have an Inner Child, and if it is suppressed or buried, it is due to the fact that you had to learn to be an adult very early on in your life. For whatever reason, you learnt that being a child was not getting you anywhere, so your survival technique was to become an adult before your childhood was complete. Here are some of thousands of reasons why this may be so:

- You were the eldest of a family where you had to be the second mum.
- You had to become the 'man' of the house.
- You were told crying got you nowhere.
- You were not wanted by your birth mother/father.
- Being seen and not being heard.
- Sexual abuse.
- Emotional abuse.
- Growing up in an unaffectionate family.
- Physical neglect.
- Growing up in a family where affection was given only on merit (development of The Pleaser and Perfectionist).
- Being born into a family where children were a sign of success of the parents or guardian.
- Being an only child.
- Learning very quickly that being a high achiever gave you attention (the beginning of the development of The Perfectionist and Pleaser).
- Having learning difficulties or physical difficulties.

Finding Your Inner Child

- Being with a family whose natural characteristics were unlike yours – being the slowest of the family or having different interests.
- Being adopted or fostered or in care.
- Having a mentally ill parent or guardian.
- Having an addictive parent or guardian (alcohol, gambling, drugs).
- An orthodox religious or strict upbringing.

THE LOVEABLE CURIOUS CHILD

The Inner Child personality is curious and inquisitive. It can't really cope with statements such as, 'What part of the word *no* don't you understand?'; 'You'll find out when you are older'; 'That's only for adults to know'. It will find that sort of communication extremely baffling and totally frustrating. The natural exploration children need when they are developing means that they will strive to understand everything; and when they can't make sense of the world, the tendency is to rebel or behave in a frustrated way.

The word 'no' brings out the child in us all; and this is another reason why food can be such an issue for people who struggle with their weight. When the adult part of you says 'no' to that second helping or something really delicious that you don't really need, The Inner Child will rebel and with its raw power overtake The Inner Adult's wishes. Your Inner Child can sometimes eat until it is physically sick.

THE WOUNDED INNER CHILD

When The Inner Child is not loved or valued and cannot make itself heard during childhood, it may well become suppressed and wounded. As a result, and in an attempt to become connected to the adult part, the only way it believes it can express itself is through primitive activities. It has so few communication skills that it will express its neediness by overindulging in food, alcohol, drugs, obsessions, promiscuity, and be drawn into bad relationships. The child part does not have the ability to become connected without the adult part becoming involved in creating that connection.

Typical emotions of the wounded child are feeling alone, being left out, not belonging, feelings of abandonment and feeling sorry for oneself. We all have these feelings from time to time, but if your Inner Child is wounded, it will take these feelings and relate them to its past, which will mean that these feelings are experienced very strongly and inappropriately. The result will be to promote low self-esteem and often depression. Depression can result when a very wounded Inner Child keeps repeating the same scenarios and experiencing the same pain, and feels helpless as they are unable to get out of the cycle they create. Some people may recognize that they have patterns in their life where they keep making wrong choices, such as choosing the wrong type of partner again and again or making the wrong choice of job or having essentially the same arguments with sisters and brothers.

A wounded Inner Child may prevent intimacy in your relationships. Your Inner Child will not be capable of enjoying love or expressing its emotions because its childhood never allowed it and it feels too dangerous. This pattern becomes an unconscious habit because, over the years, The Inner Child learns that asking for affection creates unconscious examples of rejection and embarrassment. People therefore learn very quickly: 'don't go there, you'll only get hurt'. This can be a particularly common pattern for men, hence the label 'commitment-shy'.

All children need unconditional love and affection. It is part of their developmental needs, and if it is not met, their Inner Child will be wounded.

THE FUN INNER CHILD

Once a wounded Inner Child is reconnected to your adult part, it can become childlike again. It can access all its wonderful childlike qualities and have the fun it always wanted. The list of children's traits on page 166 includes the feelings of being spontaneous, loving, open and warm. There is great satisfaction when you can laugh like a child. It's quite sad how little adults laugh and, when they do, how repressed they are when compared to the uninhibited laughter of a child.

The fun and spontaneity of childlike behaviour experienced in harmony with your adult self is refreshing. People feel they are 'more like themselves' or whole. This wholeness allows you to see the beauty of the world and to explore things unexplained through the wonderment of the child. Some people rediscover how it is to play like children play, with the innocence of a child, and find new creativity. It is very relaxing to be able to enjoy the feelings of just being, rather than doing. A child simply knows how to live in the present. They don't have high levels of anxiety about the future; they only understand now.

Nurturing Your Inner Child

When you nurture your Inner Child you can discover a wonderful internal best friend. Having an ongoing dialogue with your Inner Child can sometimes be emotional – that has the benefit of providing cathartic experiences.

> Creating the connection with your Inner Child means you can start to be a parent to yourself, rather than expecting other people to have a responsibility for you.

It means you can have much healthier relationships, personally and professionally. It also means that you can explore new experiences and take up new challenges without being stuck or prevaricating and without feeling the fear. We know that sometimes children like their routines and are suspicious of stepping out of them, so whenever you want to make a change and you feel some resistance, tell your Inner Child that it will be fun, exciting, rewarding and that you are there to make sure it is are safe. Just like with your Inner Critic, Perfectionist and Pleaser, you can have a dialogue with your child, even though the child might be hidden from you at the moment.

Once your Inner Child has been able to acknowledge that not everything always goes exactly as it would like, and that it is safe to feel whatever it is feeling because it has your support, you will flourish as a person. You will be able to laugh, cry and really enjoy who you are and know that it is safe simply to be you!

WHERE CAN I FIND MY INNER CHILD?

Take some quiet time and ask yourself the following questions:

- When was the last time you laughed till your sides split?
- When was the last time you cried?
- When was the last time you enjoyed sexual intimacy, if ever?
- How do you feel when you see two people kissing?
- When was the last time you said 'Stop the world, I'm going to have a play day'?
- When was the last time you were hugged and felt totally safe?
- When was the last time you felt you could hug and feel totally safe?
- When was the last time you had a playful fantasy day-dream?
- When did you last do something creative which was not for a purpose?
- How often can you do the above after you have consumed alcohol?

ALCOHOL AND THE INNER CHILD

Alcohol brings out your Inner Child. It is also a great way to learn about your Inner Child. We are not suggesting you go out and get drunk every night but to have a look back over your behaviour if you drink alcohol. The fascinating thing about the unsuppressed Inner Child and alcohol is that our Inner Critic, Perfectionist and Pleaser are all repressed and fall by the wayside when we drink. We do and say things we wouldn't normally; we become more sexually promiscuous, more confident, less inhibited, more intimate, more fun; and the best thing is that we say what we really feel ...

and, unfortunately, we wake the next morning to the voice of our Inner Critic demanding 'Why did you say this?', 'Why did you do that?'. Then the hurt and vulnerable child retreats until the next time you drink.

This is why some people feel they are two people: the one who is fun when they drink and the serious, boring sober person. Some people find that when they drink they become aggressive, verbally or physically, even violent. This is another way for your Inner Child to express hurt and anger, even though it is destructive to you, the adult. If you have this tendency when you drink, then you will be strongly motivated to make the connection between your Inner Child and your adult self. You are very likely to binge drink as the raw power of the child wanting to heal and be heard will be out of your control. Even without the emotional impact of your unwanted aggressive behaviour, your drinking will be doing nothing for your ability to lose excess body fat!

GET IN TOUCH WITH YOUR INNER CHILD

Ask yourself these questions. If they stir something within you, that's fine. It just indicates that your Inner Child recognizes some of these situations.

- Were your parents glad you were born?
- Were your parents able to show affection towards you?
- Were you told you were loved?
- Did either of your parents express their loving feelings towards you?
- Did your parents have open affection for each other?
- Did you feel safe to show your feelings?
- Who taught you about sex?
- Did you have friends?

- When you look back at your childhood, do you feel safe? Happy? Abandoned?
- Who did you talk to when you were scared?
- Did you have imaginary friends?
- Did you have a favourite toy?
- Did you feel like you belonged in your family?
- Did you feel like you belonged at school?
- Did you have a pet?
- Did you feel that you had any opinions?

These questions are to begin to get you in touch with your Inner Child and to explore what raw emotions are still there and suppressed within you as an adult. The feelings that are stirred are the emotions of The Inner Child, the loveable and beautiful child that gets scared, that feels pain and now wants to be healed.

Write down and complete these sentences in a place where you feel safe and secure. You can do this exercise as many times as you want as different answers may come up if you allow yourself a quiet and relaxed mind.

I remember as a child wanting so much to ....
If I could be there for my Inner Child now, I would say to him/her ....
I used to get into trouble because I was ....
Growing up I felt ....
When I was a child I promised myself I would always be ....
When I was a child I wanted to grow up and be ....
I really admired .... for being so ....
When I was lonely I would ....
When I was happy I would ....
The games I most liked to play were ....
My most favourite thing was ....

The best thing I can remember about school was.............................
The worst thing I can remember about school was.............................

HOW TO TALK TO YOUR INNER CHILD

Find a time during your day when you can talk to your Inner Child. This
time needs to be set, as children like consistency. Keep to the commitment.
You may choose a walk in the park or sitting down in a quiet room,
whatever scenario that allows your Inner Child to feel safe. Some people
like to sit their imaginary child on their lap or hold hands. Perhaps you
have a picture of yourself as a child, so you can physically have an image
of yourself. Start to talk to your Inner Child like you would to a child with
a basic understanding of language. You can ask questions such as:

- How are you feeling today?
- Is there anything this week that made you feel good?
- Is there anything this week that made you feel sad?
- What person do you feel really safe with?
- What person do you feel unsafe with?
- Are you happy?
- If no, why do you feel unhappy?
- What makes you feel happy?
- What makes you feel angry?
- Can you remember your favourite book?
- Can you remember your favourite film?
- If you need help, who do you turn to?
- If you need unconditional love, how do you express it?
- Where do you feel the most safe?

Spend this time each day asking questions like these, so you can start to learn about what your Inner Child likes and needs, and how to make it feel loved and safe. Talk to your Inner Child as if it is real, because your Inner Child is real. Each of us was a child, even if it seems like a long time ago! This powerful part is as real as The Inner Critic, The Pleaser etc.

It is recommended that you use a very quiet time, when you are in a state of self-hypnosis, to imagine the following scene. You can use your own words:

> Look into your Inner Child's eyes and tell them they are safe and that it is OK now to talk without judgement, without anger and without hurt. Tell your Inner Child that it is safe to speak out now and that you are sorry it has taken such a long time to talk. Tell them that you didn't know how to talk before and from now on that you, the adult, the inner parent, will look after them. Tell them that it is important to understand that you have the ability now to listen and learn and reconnect with your Inner Child, that they have finally come home. Tell them that you will try your best to make them feel safe and warm, and when life gets scary you will be there to protect your Inner Child like no other parent could ever have done. Hug each other and promise each other that, whenever they get scared, you will be there. Tell them that it is safe to cry and that it is safe to be angry or sad, and that they can talk to you about it whenever they want. Tell them that they are not responsible for their parents' relationship with each other; that they are not responsible for any family problems they have experienced. Tell them how much you love them and that they don't need to overeat or drink too much anymore because their needs are being met by talking and making them feel safe. Explain that food is something that belongs to how your Inner Child used to feel and it is safe to let

go of those thoughts, feelings and behaviours. Tell them that you now have each other and will always have each other. Tell your Inner Child that it is now safe to be safe and to be able to be the fun, happy child that children all deserve to be. That, finally, they are home and that they are a very special child who deserves infinite love and support.

John's Story

John was not progressing very well on the Slim by Suggestion programme. He was pooh-poohing the whole emotional part. In fact, we were surprised that he kept coming back to see us.

John, a taxi driver, was happily married with three children. He was quite aggressive, and a number of people felt the need to tell him so gently during the assertiveness skills session. When we came to The Inner Child section, we (being therapists) were aware that this would probably stir a lot inside John, and we were right. John did not stay for the hypnosis section that evening, which was very unusual. In fact, we thought we wouldn't see him again. However, John phoned a few days later and said that he wanted to see one of us for a one-to-one private appointment. We were delighted.

John came to Georgia and was very tense. Once he sat down, the tears started to flow. He said that The Inner Child section had brought up too many memories of his childhood, a childhood he felt was not a happy one. He explained that his father used to hit him when he was drunk and that he had never had an affectionate relationship with either parent. His mother was too busy avoiding the fact that her child was being hurt, and everything was swept under the carpet.

John then went on to say that the only way he could protect himself emotionally at school was to be a tough, unemotional guy.

He made fun of weak, insipid children. He stirred up lots of physical fights and was constantly in trouble with the teachers. This, in turn, led to more beatings at home.

I explained to John that he had done the best he possibly could with the resources he had been given, and that being the tough guy was the only way he knew how to protect himself physically against people his own size, and also emotionally. After some exploration, we discovered that he associated being slim with being punished as his mother used to send him to bed without any dinner most days of the week. He felt very angry with everybody and with himself, so we undertook some Inner Child work.

John now says that he feels like he has lost four stone in his brain and that at last he can be a much better father and husband.

Never underestimate the power of your Inner Child.
Don't ignore it. If you do, it will become destructive because it needs attention.

Eileen's Story

Eileen was a very quiet participant on the programme. She didn't really give any input to the group discussions as she behaved very passively and shyly. When we discussed The Inner Child, she became very tearful. During the hypnosis, she moved into a foetal position and cried quietly.

Tears may be experienced during this type of work and this is always a cathartic experience. Eileen felt very embarrassed and was extremely apologetic after the hypnosis. We explained that her experience was normal and that it is far better to let the tears flow than to hold them back. Whenever you feel like crying, just remember that tears are always 'better out than in'. If you prevent yourself from crying and experiencing the emotion, even when it is tears of joy, you will be repressing something. When you repress something you are still going to have to deal with it later.

The next week, Eileen came in and was quite playful and witty. She said she had completed all the exercises in this book and now finally felt some sense of closure and inner peace. Eileen said she recognized that she had been avoiding intimate moments with her husband and dreaded to be touched or to make love. She and her husband had not really had a sexual relationship for many years, and during that time she had piled on the weight to protect her Inner Child from being touched. Eileen felt that healing her Inner Child meant she could have fun again and laugh and start to become more sexual and physical.

There were obviously things she needed to address with her husband concerning their relationship. However, Eileen recognized that part of the healing of her Inner Child was simply that it is safe to be held, it is safe to be loved and it is safe to have loving touch.

Six months later, Roz saw Eileen. She was quite glowing with self-confidence and her weight had dropped by two stone. She said, 'Out of all the things I learnt on the programme and through the CD, it was the Inner Child stuff that really allowed me to be me.'

SOME THINGS TO TRY

There are many exercises within this chapter that can be repeated, together with listening to Track 4 on your CD. You can also try spending some quality time with your child part. It will give you an added dimension to your leisure time, guaranteed!

How long is it since you felt the experience of living life NOW, with no concern for past or present, just experiencing? When was the last time you spent the afternoon exploring or pottering around? How often do you go to a funny movie and really laugh? How often do you set aside quality time to be intimate with your partner? How often do you walk in the park and look at how beautiful the trees and flowers are? Many of you won't be able to remember the last time!

Set aside time twice a week when you are simply 'being', not doing. It takes practice but your Inner Child will be so thankful that you could share this feeling. It may be difficult to make the time, but with a little practice you will enjoy yourself so much that you will want to set aside time regularly to experience living without the adult necessity to 'do' or achieve something.

13
Completing the Programme and Your Inner Adviser

You have now come to the end of the seventh week of the programme. Once you have read this chapter, you need to spend just another six to seven days listening to Track 4 on your CD. After this, you will have finished the official 10-step Slim by Suggestion programme. Congratulations! You will be feeling lighter mentally and physically, and you know you can keep the motivation to stay on the Slim by Suggestion programme for as long as it takes to achieve the body size you desire.

It's our experience that from about week six, participants on the programme seem to feel that the weeks have flown by, and often comment that they wonder what it will be like when the programme finishes. By now, participants are feeling good about themselves, and realize that they have much more confidence – around food, about themselves and in their relationships with other people. Good self-esteem is a really important facet of the programme as it is what everybody needs when they want to make and maintain positive change. The CD tracks are very important, along with personal exploration through your Emotional Journal, in creating that high self-esteem. All 10 steps and the contents of the chapters are about making and maintaining that positive change and allowing the slim part to come forward and take its rightful place.

What is Self-esteem?

One of the core aims of the programme is providing you with the mind tools to gain control over your thinking. By doing so, you establish control over your emotions and your behaviours. The result of this is confidence, which we call self-confidence. 'Self-esteem' is when you use your thinking skills effectively – that's because you will feel good in yourself and in control of your behaviours without having to monitor them. You will feel like a 'whole' person.

> With self-esteem, you will find that feeling good, enthusiastic and full of life is your normal state of mind.

There are some things you need to know and look out for in relation to self-esteem. On the positive side, you will easily maintain high levels of self-esteem by encouraging positive self-talk, having effective negotiations with your Inner Dialogue, and you will know that your emotions and behaviour are stable. On the less positive side, self-esteem can get dented by events in your life, and before you know it consciously, you may find one or two of the foundations of good self-esteem being gradually eroded. It goes back to the functioning of the unconscious mind. If a relationship fails, your work appraisal didn't go to plan or you had a tiny binge, your confidence can be temporarily dented. However, strong protective mechanisms may kick in as these type of events make you feel vulnerable. If this happens, then all the protective parts attempt to get heard and your emotions and behaviour may become unstable. Because you have been through the 10 steps of the Slim by Suggestion programme, you will know how to recognize this and you will know what to do.

It's all about recognizing what went on: did events trigger old emotions? Were you physically tired and reacted to events with stress? Did you get manipulated as you didn't behave assertively? Did a family thing bring up angry feelings? Did this result in you pushing things down with food or drink? Whatever happened, it's just a lapse, not a collapse. Just bear in mind that self-esteem is not a static entity; it can go up as well as down. All you have to do is be aware of events and their effects and take action if you need to.

Maintaining the Programme and Your Self-esteem

If you need to take action to enhance your self-esteem, all you need to do is listen to your CD, reread the chapter or chapters that seem relevant and take time to use your Emotional Journal. It's about being nice to yourself and taking some quality time to get back on track. It can be helpful to re-evaluate yourself too:

- After six months, redo the questionnaires and consider the answers and what they are indicating to you. How do they compare, and is there a particular aspect that has changed? You can reread the relevant notes in Chapter 6 and take action.

- If you find that you are slipping back into old habits, you will have to address the fact that you may not have worked though everything on the programme and there is a block or issue that you have not tackled. It is likely to be the very thing that you do not want to tackle and you will need to use the CD and your Emotional Journal to unearth whatever it is that is deeply buried in your unconscious mind. Using the CD is important as it will enable you to safely deal with the trigger unconsciously, and you will only have to be aware of the effects on your behaviour and change that behaviour.

- Are you really eating a healthy diet? Reassess what it is you are eating. You might find that unnecessary items are creeping into your healthy-eating programme and you need a boost with Tracks 1 and 2 of your CD. Use the Healthy-living Diary method to see exactly what you are eating and drinking.

- Are you eating when you are not hungry? You will need to tackle this with all the mind tools you have gained on the programme and use the CD to motivate yourself, as well as taking the steps outlined in the points above.

- Different life stages can also be challenging: the man who retires or gets made redundant; the woman who is approaching menopause; a fit person who has to exercise less for a physical reason; when children leave home. Circumstances are not static and there are fresh challenges at every life stage. You will need to re-evaluate yourself and see if there are old beliefs around your new circumstances that have only just surfaced. Rereading the chapters that seem relevant will be helpful, along with using the Emotional Journal and the CD.

Introducing Your Inner Adviser

There is another mind tool that many people find useful. We call it The Inner Adviser. This helps to create further self-reliance and self-sufficiency, and is a tool you can use to maintain self-esteem. Its other benefits are:

- It will guide you out of a negative state.
- It will provide you with internal unconditional support, no matter what is going on in your life.
- It will be there for you when you need to make a decision but cannot seem to choose between all the options running through your mind.
- It will be there for you when other people are trying to sway you towards doing things their way.
- It provides support to keep you on track and motivated, or when things get difficult.
- Your Inner Adviser will always show you that you can get there; you have the unconscious tools to achieve your goals.
- When you are stuck in a dilemma and no solution comes to mind, your Inner Adviser will guide you.
- An Inner Adviser means that you will be able to rely on your own feelings, thoughts and actions, rather than waiting for a friend, a partner or a parent to give you guidance. You will give yourself your own answers to your own thoughts, and this means that your relationship with other people will dramatically improve.
- Your Inner Adviser is a great tool to use when you are planning your goals.

- Having a strong Inner Adviser will allow you to see that you do have choices and you do have the strength to do what is right for you.
- When people have educated themselves to listen to their Inner Adviser, they will not need to rely on anybody else to make a decision for them. This immediately allows you to become more independent, more confident and have a feeling of internal safety. This self-sufficient feeling also means that one intuitive decision can lead to others. Each time you act on an intuitive decision, it creates an unconscious habit to trust yourself.
- For some people, connecting with their Inner Adviser feels like coming home. After all, when we were little, most of us had an imaginary friend or a toy that talked to us that nobody else could hear. Your Inner Adviser is just like that very special friend.

WHAT IS AN INNER ADVISER?

Your Inner Adviser can be described as your special friend or as a thinking tool. Yet it is more than that as it is the most intuitive part within you. It is so powerful and yet so often overlooked, or should we say 'underheard'. How many times do we ask ourselves a question, hear our own answer, then do the opposite – what other people want us to do? Then we get cross and The Inner Critic can say, 'Why didn't you act on your own advice?'

Your Inner Adviser is the voice that can help you make the right decision for you, not the decision you think you should make. It's the part that can advise you with only your best interests at heart, as it knows all about you. Some people think of it as their own mentor.

Your Inner Adviser can also act as someone different to you, and can let you know how that person would act in any situation. For instance, if you are standing at a buffet, barbecue or any other eating occasion and you are tempted to indulge, you can ask your Inner Adviser, 'How would Jane Fonda, Tiger Woods, Venus Williams, Madonna [any role model who maintains a fit and trim figure] deal with this situation?' Your Inner Adviser will be able to give you the answer – and it won't sound like you; it will sound wiser and give you advice or guidance that you would not have thought of for yourself. Some people find their Inner Adviser can imitate other people's voices; some people find their Adviser will create a visual image of a suggested solution.

Some of you reading this will think it quite mad, but just try it and see. It might seem mad – but if it is a tool you find useful, why not use it?

Your Inner Adviser has always been with you. Some people will recognize The Inner Adviser as the part that just pops up without conscious thought when they need to make any decision. This is because of the sequence of events that takes place when we scan our minds for information. The mind will look for instances of previous experiences and how you behaved and felt in a similar situation, and the answer will come. However, you now know that this answer may not be accurate or what you want anymore. Some people's Inner Adviser may intervene and give them a more appropriate scenario. Remember, the unconscious mind will always refer to what it has experienced first, rather than the new experience or idea. That is why an Inner Adviser can help you move out of the constant cycle of old patterns that you want to leave behind. If you aren't connected to your Inner Adviser yet, you will be able to do so with practice.

Many people who have strong Pleasers will have difficulty making a decision for themselves because they have a tendency to worry about what other people think. If you have a strong Pleaser, you may not even have thought about what you really want.

In fact, humans, no matter how strong or weak their Pleaser part, do tend to be driven by what other people think, to comply with the values their particular society has decided upon. This leads us down a path where we cross-reference our thoughts and actions externally as, broadly speaking, we are taught to listen to other people before making a decision for ourselves. This becomes a habit, and so before we take action we think about what other people would do or think. This is a bit like having an Inner Censor or an Inner Judgmental part. This can and will undermine your resolve, confuse and discourage you and erode your self-esteem, which you need to keep going on your healthy-eating programme.

Most people have, through their background and education, suppressed The Inner Adviser. The reasons can be:

- being unable to express yourself freely as a child
- being ridiculed for having an imaginary friend as a child
- time spent in the company of judgmental people
- lack of self-belief (self-esteem)
- one bad decision leading to procrastination and inability to move on
- fear of change
- fear of success or its companion, fear of failure

Some people get to a point when they are not sure what they want in a particular area of their life, such as relationships, work or life in general.

Slim by Suggestion

They will have asked the advice of all their friends, colleagues, family etc. The problem with this is that they are not satisfied with the answers from other people; they just don't feel 'right'. Their own suppressed Inner Adviser is trying to be heard and they will feel anxiety and disquiet. Their intuition is saying something is not right and the solutions or decisions suggested are not the best ones for them. We know how powerful the unconscious mind is when it wants to protect you. Some people get ill and some become anxious, whatever it takes to stop them going down the 'wrong' path.

Sometimes they force themselves into taking an intuitively 'wrong' decision and then feel guilt, regret and mistrust themselves. These feelings then create low self-worth, negative beliefs and depression, and can lead to unwanted behaviour around food.

When you cross-reference externally using family, friends and colleagues, it is wonderful to know that they want to help. However, in every case, their choices and advice reflect their own internal fears and beliefs rather than yours, so relying on others can be a poor strategy.

Other people do see the world differently. There will always be people who will try and sway you towards their way of thinking, so it is wise to be careful. There are many saboteurs out there – who have great delight in trying to convince you that you can eat that second helping. That sort of friend is jealous that you have made a decision and you want to stick to it. Saboteurs come in all shapes and sizes: mums, dads, boyfriends, girlfriends, work colleagues. You may think they are trying to be supportive or that they are trying to help, but be careful. If you have people around who behave in that way, you can be sure your Inner Adviser has been trying to let you know for a long time. As you read this, you may call to mind a particular person; you may feel a stirring inside. If so, the chances are that this person is not helping you; they are trying to feel better about themselves, and when you eat that second helping, you will feel worse about yourself. That's a good result for a saboteur.

Completing the Programme

HOW TO CONNECT TO YOUR INNER ADVISERS

There are many techniques for connecting to your Inner Adviser(s). We've listed them in random order:

- You can use time during your self-hypnosis/listening to your CD. When you drift into your own inner world, you can ask for your Inner Adviser to come forward. Some visual people do 'meet' an image. It could be someone you know, such as a grandparent or other significant adult from your past. For others, it is a fictitious/imagined wise old man or woman. Sometimes a picture or photograph of someone comes to life. Sometimes it is you, but with a different and wiser ego; this is normally called your Higher Self, the self that is most connected to your soul. Others will hear a voice that is not theirs, and some people just experience feelings and sensations. In any event, you can ask, silently and mentally, for solutions to your dilemma. Ask how to deal with a situation; ask for advice. You can really ask for anything and any question, and you will get an answer. It may come some time later or immediately. It may not be the answer you wanted to hear and the answer may come to you in an unexpected way – for example, as a signal or a sign that is meaningful to you and that you understand.
- You can lie still and quietly relax into a light trance. Rehearse your goals of the future and ask your Inner Adviser to assist you to create what is really right for you.
- You might want to have a brainstorming session with collection of Advisers. Say you have a problem that is creating

stress and unwanted eating because you can't find a solution. You could sit and relax, imagine all the successful people you admire and bring them to your brainstorming session. Some people have a business meeting with them in their imagination; others have a social meeting where everybody has a chance to come up with the right solution for you. It's your imagination so you can have who or whatever you want in your mind. It's your call!

- Just giving yourself the space to ask for help means you are open to it. As they say, if you don't ask, you won't get. So start asking questions. Ask for motivation. You will gain self-esteem when you refer internally rather than externally.

Jane's Story

Jane and her partner were always frustrated that she could never make her own decisions. Whenever she had to decide on something, she would always consult other people. It was almost a compulsion and it certainly was a habit. She discovered that her belief system was 'other people's decisions are always better than mine'. Once she realized it was her belief system that was holding her back, she then created Inner Advisers in her mind. One was her own and the rest were other people. This allowed her to feel safe about making decisions without actually asking others and looking outside herself for the answers.

As a result, it allowed her to be much more independent and confident about her own life. Jane was surprised to find that after practising this in her own mind it became second nature and she had developed a new and useful habit.

Jane has since been promoted to a position everybody knew she could handle and she is delighted. Her relationship with her partner is much better. He is more relaxed knowing that she does not rely on him emotionally all the time.

Katie's Story

Katie came on the Slim by Suggestion programme two months prior to her holiday in Spain. She wanted to look her best and, after years of yo-yo dieting, made the decision that the programme was her only and last resort. She was very shy and lacked assertiveness skills. She was habitually unable to make a decision, so attending the programme was a big commitment for her. Katie really enjoyed the CD and listened to it daily. She saw results as she went from being size 16 to size 14 over the eight weeks.

She told us that because she had started to take responsibility for herself via her Inner Adviser, she felt so supported that it didn't matter what happened; she was able to feel as if she belonged to herself. She said, 'I felt for the first time in my life that I had someone who knew me so well, who will direct me towards what I want rather than just doing what I thought others wanted.'

Katie also said that it was the first time in her life she had truly looked forward to going on holiday. Previously she had dreaded the 'beach scene', surrounded by her slim friends, and the evenings out where she felt totally inadequate, physically and emotionally. She was also able to recognize that some of her friends were saboteurs, and that her Inner Adviser/intuition had been trying to tell her this for some time. She said that she finally felt she had a mind tool to help her deal with her shyness. Katie finally felt she belonged and had a mind of her own.

Be sure you have thought through your personal, physical and professional goals (*see Chapter 9*). Then set about gaining the advice you need from yourself.

- Write down all the things you have thought about doing, even if you don't think they are possible. Your list could include ideas such as abseiling, painting, writing, travelling, leaving your job, making a daunting career change. Now sit and think about your list. Does it stir up fear or anxiety? Do you feel uncomfortable? Your belief system causes this stirred-up feeling because you have learnt that you 'can't' do these things. Use your Inner Adviser(s) to help.
- Test out your Inner Adviser the very next time you have to come to a decision or you feel stuck. You will have a surprising experience!

As You Complete the Programme ...

In six to seven days, you will have completed the Slim by Suggestion programme. You can feel very proud of yourself. It is now time to redo your questionnaires from Chapter 6. Don't be tempted to look at your previous answers until you have completed the questionnaires for the second time. Many people will have made big changes and will be able to gauge them from their scores. Those who scored within the 'normal' range when they first completed the questionnaires and who may not see significant shifts will be able to look at how their behaviour around food has changed and how they are much more in control in so many areas of their lives.

For everyone, just think about your confidence levels and how you think and feel about eating and drinking in comparison with how you felt just eight weeks ago. From now on, you will always be able to recognize when your Inner Dialogue, your emotions and your behaviour are not as you would wish, and you have all of the Slim by Suggestion techniques and tools to use to keep you slim, motivated and confident.

Slim by Suggestion

Bibliography and Further Reading

Aston, Donna. *Fat or Fiction*, Hybrid, 1999

Black, Jack. *Mindstore*, Thorsons, 1994

Bradshaw, John. *Homecoming*, Piatkus, 1990

Briffa, Dr John. Body Wise, Cima, 2000

Brookes, David. *Beat Stress From Within*, Hollanden Publishing Ltd., 1997

Buzan, Tony. *Make the Most of Your Mind*, BBC, 1988

Buzan, Tony. *Use your Head*, BBC, 1997

Glenville, Marilyn. *Natural Alternatives to Dieting*, Kyle Cathie Ltd., 1999

Hill, Napoleon. *Think and Grow Rich*, Wilshire Book Co., 1937

Jeffers, Susan. *Feel the Fear and do it Anyway*, Arrow, 1991

Johnson, Rex and Swindley, David. *Creating Confidence*, Element, 1994

Maltz, Maxwell. *Psychocybernetics*, Wilshire Book Co., 1960

Maltx, Maxwell. *Psycho-Cybernetics 2000*, Wilshire Books, 1997

Laroque, Dr Maurice. *Slim Within*, Bariatrix International Inc., 1989

Lindenfield, Gael. *Managing Anger*, Thorsons, London, 1993

Powell, Trevor J. and Enright, Simon J. *Anxiety and Stress Management*, Routledge, London, 1982

Rees, Shan and Graham, Roderick S. *Assertion Training – How To Be Who You Really Are*, Routledge, London, 1991

Stone, Hal and Winkelman, Sidra. *Embracing Our Selves*, Nataraj Publishing, 1989

Stone, Hal and Sidra. *Embracing the Inner Critic*, HarperSanFrancisco, 1993

Talley, P. Forrest. *Psychotherapy Research and Practice, Bridging the Gap*, Basic Books, 1995

Tribole, Evelyn and Resch, Elyse. *Intuitive Eating*, St Martin's Press, New York, 1995

Working Effectively – Managing Stress Workbook, The Open College for the National Extension College, Cambridge, 1997

Yapko, Dr Michael. *Breaking the Patterns of Depression*, Doubleday, 1997

Yapko, Dr Michael. *Essentials of Hypnosis*, Brunner Mazel, 1995

Resources

Slim by Suggestion hosts regular workshops. For more information, see our website on www.slimbysuggestion.com

Replacement Slim By Suggestion CDs and the most up-to-date versions can also be obtained through our website.